Happy Twin Mum

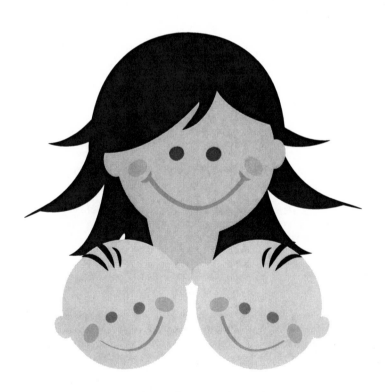

Supportive ideas for the first three years

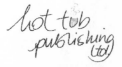

Happy Twin Mum ISBN 978-0-9576753-2-2
First published 2013 in Great Britain

Hot Tub Publishing Limited., EX1 1BR, Exeter, Devon, UK
info@hottubpublishingltd.co.uk

Happy
Twin Mum

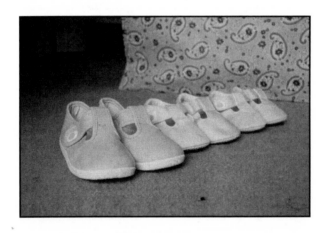

DEDICATION

Dedicated to my children;
may all your dreams come true.

CONTENTS

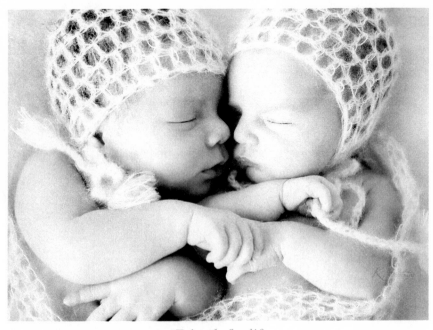

Friends for life

INTRODUCTION

One egg, two eggs, IVF or SEX, boys, girls or one of each - who cares? The result is the same: you are holding two babies and you have an incredible journey ahead of you!

Having two babies is an amazing and very special event that without a doubt has the power to turn life as you know it upside down. Suddenly there are (another) two little people on this planet who depend on you, need you and unconditionally love you but at the same time are taking up pretty much all of your time, communicate by crying and rob you of your sleep. The first years even with just one baby are quite a journey, with two babies it's an expedition into the wild! I wanted to be prepared for this expedition and enjoy every step of the way. I knew my babies would be born early and that we would have to stay in neonatal care. I had a child already and was going to be holding two bundles of joy plus a three year old bundle of fun and I was wondering what I could do to make sure I would be able to completely enjoy my three young children, my husband and myself? The answer was mainly by keeping periods of feeling overwhelmed and exhausted at bay, by getting organised and by feeling good about myself.

It's exciting to become a mother, no matter how many children, but many mothers experience Supermum Exhaustion as I like to call it. Of course, hormones play a role but other factors such as lack of sleep and reduced socialising play an important role too. I believe some feelings build up unnoticed long before you experience the effects - but how to avoid the potholes?

I certainly didn't want to feel overwhelmed and exhausted, so I took a closer look at areas I could influence and structured everything into ten chapters, one for each of the key areas I had found:

1. Help

2. Socialising and Support

3. Sleep

4. Coping with crying

5. Confidence with feeding

6. Managing your new family life

7. Healthy self expectations

8. Realistic relationship expectations

9. The birth and a stay in the neonatal care unit

10. Life with additional needs

Having twins is great but it can be hard work at times as the little stories told in this book will show. There are a million funny stories to be told too, the reason you find the more challenging ones here instead is done with the aim to reassure that you are not the only one when you find yourself in the midst of twinland madness.

I didn't write this book to scare any expectant twin parents, but at the same time there's no point in pretending that all will be easy. I published this book as I believe that what helped me, can help you to prevent yourself from feeling low and exhausted. Some parts of the book might appear a little "over the top" during pregnancy, but six months later when in the midst of having two little babies they might offer valuable support.

I have no intention of rewriting and rephrasing twin publications already available, I won't be telling you what buggy to buy or how many vests to put in your hospital bag. My only aim was to write a feel good you are not alone book, a book to help you enjoy yourself, your twins, any siblings and your partner when things get a bit hectic. And I want this book to be your friend, the friend who has twins too, and who knows what it's like when you wish you were an octopus because two arms just aren't enough.

This might be the biggest challenge of your life; it might even push you to your limits. However, it's an incredible experience and it's important to remember that every day is a gift and every challenging day offers an opportunity to help your babies develop into happy and trusting individuals.

Once you return from your expedition into baby-twinland you will have learned so much about yourself, you will be way more laid back than you have ever been and you will have a great time ahead with two toddling comedians.

Enjoy yourself, your two babies and the rest of your family.

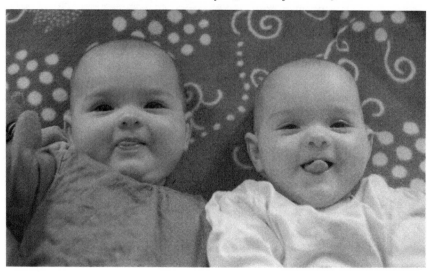

ABOUT ME

My name is Kerri, my son Jacob was three years old when his sisters Jess and Isla were born. I live in the UK with my husband Rich.

It was whilst I was expecting that I crafted a plan on how to keep exhaustion and feeling overwhelmed at bay and this plan became my passion for the following three years. I kept a diary, spoke to hundreds of mothers of twins, interviewed many of them and quizzed health professionals. I read every twin book I could grab hold of, I read a lot about postnatal depression (PND) and visited a support group for challenged mothers. I read (too) many parenting books, became chair of my local twins club, became a facilitator for the Twins and Multiple Births Foundation (TAMBA) and basically spent every spare minute on this project, and half way through I realised that I was actually in the midst of writing a book.

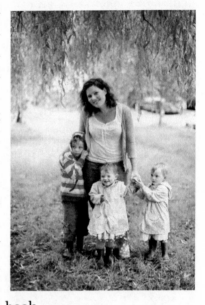

This might sound like I am Superwoman, I am not! Having twins didn't come easy and I didn't really have a lot of time to write a book, I am just really passionate about this project. I invested every spare minute in it and I loved it. Many of the sources I refer to are UK based but they are accessible and useful regardless of where you are in the world.

When my girls were little I didn't get the chance to type on the computer so I simply wrote on anything I could find. On two occasions it was loo roll. Sometimes I just recorded my thoughts with my phone. This isn't a guide on what to do or not to do, it's a collection of thoughts, stories and strategies - they worked for me and they might work for you. I simply care for other mums and feel that sharing my experiences has the potential to help others.

This is a book for mothers of twins and as much as I would have liked it to be for fathers too, I must admit that due to the fact that it's based on my own experiences, it will not cover all aspects concerning a father of twins.

Many chapters contain additional info for parents of older siblings. Look out for the icon on the left. I have added a "glimpse into the future" at the end of some chapters, to demonstrate that things really will get easier!

Life with two babies is exciting and challenging, one day you will cope just fine, other days you might feel exhausted. That's the way it goes.

You don't want to be wishing time away but sometimes you might feel like it's just "never ending" and during those moments it helps to know that it will get easier once those dependent little babies turn into toddling, chattering little people. It will remain a challenge but very different to the challenge of having two babies, more entertaining and less draining.

ABOUT YOU

You are amazing! Your body has been home to two babies, they have grown inside YOUR body and you dedicated your body to those two little people. Your body has physically been serving those two little lives for several months; you have looked after them, worried about them, cared for them and given birth to them.

You have achieved something amazing!

Your days are most likely dedicated to the care of your babies, so are your nights. This is a 24/7, 100% dedication job and you are so lucky to have landed it! Now is not the time to think that you can't go out as much as you used to, that your body looks different, that your favourite dress no longer fits and that your once so immaculate house looks like a bomb has hit – that's just not what life is about at the moment!

Enjoy yourself, don't put yourself under too much pressure, be realistic and enjoy this precious time with those tiny creatures, even though the baby stage might seem never ending at times, the fact is it will fly by and you will really regret it if all you remember is how much you have whinged about yourself. In ten years time you won't have fond memories of a clean kitchen and how you starved yourself back into that size silly dress, instead you will remember your baby twins lying bare bottomed on the change mat, wriggling their chubby bodies whilst you're singing along to Kylie Minogue's "All The Lovers..."

{CHAPTER 1}

HELP

"That's better," said the sonographer.
"Now I can see them both. You're expecting twins."
"Help!" was one of my first thoughts, quickly followed by
"How lucky am I?"

The question as to whether help will be needed or not seems to be one of the first questions for many expectant twin mums, hence I decided to dedicate the first chapter to this very question. Let's start this book with some good news for those with no help to hand; it can be done without help, even if you have older children: You can do it!

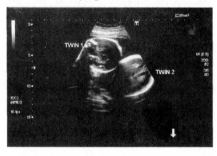

When I first found out I was expecting twins, I didn't have a clue what to expect but I was a little worried that I might have a rather busy time ahead with a three year old and two babies. I am generally up for any challenge and battle my way through by myself, and my little sister often warns me: "Take it easy! You are not King Kong Kerri."

So this time I thought I was being ever so sensible and organised a cleaner for the first few weeks after birth. But what other help would I need? Would I need any help at all?

A few years on and I have come to realise that I had been asking myself the wrong question. I should have asked myself: "Will I want help?" instead and the answer would have been a straight forward "YES"!

There will be times when things get a bit hectic and you can simply do with a helping hand, may it be for an hour or a whole day, when you appreciate a break, a little sleep, some company or an actual (semi) adult conversation.

During the last few years I have been asking hundreds of multiple mums about what sort of help they appreciate and it gave me the idea of compiling THE TWIN FRIEND HELP LIST. It will help you identify what help you might appreciate and it helps yourw friends and family to see that there are lots of different ways of helping other than babysitting, which can seem a daunting task to some. Remember that no one is "useless" and anyone can do something to help you as the next pages will show. You can download a copy of the TWIN FRIEND HELP LIST from my website www.lifewithtwins.co.uk or create your own and hand the list to your friends and family, it will help them to help you! Or you could even take it a step further: When you get married you have bridesmaids to help you with all the preparations and during the big day. Having two babies is a much bigger event than a wedding, so why not choose a twin-maid of honour, create a personal help-list, just like you would have a gift list at a wedding, and get your twin-maid of honour to distribute and oversee the list.

If you don't feel you could give the list to any of your friends and family, read it regardless as it might give you some ideas on how to organise any help when it's offered.

If you don't have any potential help, don't worry - finding help is even easier once your babies have arrived and people actually see that you have your hands quite full. You can still rope in new helpers later on, as the pages following the list will demonstrate.

THE TWIN FRIEND HELP-LIST

Hi all, I bought a book called "Happy Twin Mum" and the author Kerri Miller suggests to be brave and hand out the list below to friends and family in order to make it easier to help and support our family.

• When you visit, always get a little job done: hang up the laundry, fold dry laundry, empty and reload the dish washer, take out the rubbish or grab the vacuum cleaner, duster or broom and just get a little bit done, it doesn't take long and makes a big difference.

• Do little jobs that require leaving the house such as taking out the rubbish, sorting the recycling, taking bins or recycling to the road, unloading shopping from the car, posting letters, popping out to the shop or pharmacy.

• If the babies are asleep, ask the twin parents if they would like to have a nap or a shower whilst you listen out for the babies. Or ask the twin parents what job they would try and get done now if they were on their own and then go on to do the job together with them.

• Don't stay too long, unless you continue to do something helpful and let the twin parent carry on with what they need to do.

• If one baby is asleep and you seem to be doing fine with the other (you are now down to a very manageable one adult one baby ratio) offer the twin parent the chance to have a shower, nap, check their emails etc.

• Whenever you plan a visit, please check in advance if they need anything like bread or milk etc, a quick text message before you leave is all it takes.

• Make a drink for everyone.

- Cook dinner for the new twin parents during their first weeks at home, simply cook during the day in your own kitchen, wrap it up oven ready and drop it off. Organise this together with other friends.

- Take the twins and other children for a walk and give mum or dad a break.

- Come in during "meltdown" times such as dinner time, bath time and bed time. Even just half an hour per week makes a huge difference. If the babies are bottle fed plan your visit so that you can help with at least one feed.

- Thinking of cancelling a visit? Don't! Unless you really have to and then cancel as early as possible. Same for delays: If you're going to be late, let them know!

- Keeping company is also a form of helping!

- When the babies have started solids, bring baby food! Either cook a batch or buy some pots, pouches or jars. It's always comforting for a twin parent to have some spare sat on the shelf or in the freezer.

- Offer to come along to baby clinics, doctors or hospital appointments, twins club, swimming lessons, soft play areas, playgrounds or toddler groups. Meet in a park, forest etc, which is great in order to get everyone out of the house. You could come to their house first and help load up the kids, buggy and the one million bags and help to remember everything they might need. Or you could offer to come along to do the weekly shop. Having a baby each in your shopping trolley will save having to answer all the lovingly meant but very time consuming twin-questions.

THANK YOU FOR HELPING!

FINDING HELP

Some of us have only a few friends and family members around who could help and I found myself in this situation. My family live too far away to help and most of my friends have little children of their own. Luckily my in-laws lived just down the road and during pregnancy this seemed to be the only (but most amazing) help I would have.

Well, I was wrong. A few months down the line and I had plenty of help, I was holding the golden tickets to finding help in my arms – my twins, two babies, and an incredibly cute three year old of course. I made so many new friends. People feel happy to help with twins; you just have to invite these people into your life! Maybe some of the things I did, which I will explain in just a minute, might give you an idea. Or you could visit your local twins club and ask other twin mums what help they have had, they might know about some local scheme or pass your details on.

Some make the conscious decision not to accept or seek any help and I spoke to many twin mums who did it by themselves with no help at all, or just help frowm their partners in the evenings, and of course that's possible. You can do it on your own; even with older siblings, but having been there I feel that it can be much healthier and way more fun to accept help every now and then. You might feel like you don't need or want any help right now but at least take the potential helper's phone number if offered. You never know, things might just

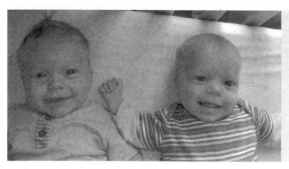

Who wouldn't want to offer help with these cuties: three months olds Sacha and Barnaby.

change all of a sudden and it is a comforting feeling knowing that there is someone who you could call on. Let me introduce my little help network:

I organised a volunteer

There are charities out there offering help by sending a volunteer to your house for a set number of hours every week. I contacted the UK charity Home Start and soon was sent a volunteer to help. The first attempt didn't work out at all but my second volunteer, Barbara, was lovely and such a great help. I really enjoyed those three hours every week when she came to our house and played with the kids whilst I had a quick shower or prepared dinner. She took the girls for a walk so I could spend time with Jacob, or she came into town with us. She stayed on for about four months until the girls were nearly one year old.

I made friends with (preferably pre-party-age) teenage girls who love babies / little children

Demands for help change quite a lot throughout the first couple of years, just like our babies do. The teenage girl across the road didn't seem like a suitable help when my babies were tiny and fragile but once they got to the age where they liked a bit of entertainment, the same teenager was just perfect to keep the children happy whilst I did a few chores or prepared their food. I had the help of Kathryn (then 16, whose granny lives across the road) and Emma (then 17, who lives just round the corner and kindly offered her help when I bumped into her) and they have been amazing and as an added bonus I am now that Ed Sheeran is 'totally hot' and I also know every detail about the Twilight Saga and Robert Pattinson's love life!

They took the babies for a walk, chased Jacob round the house, came over to help at dinner time, helped to bath the babies and also any time when they had nothing else to do;

they knew they were always welcome to come over and spend time with us. Both of them applied for the Duke of Edinburgh's Award and volunteering was part of achieving the award. A win –win situation!

One lady at twins club approached a nearby nursing college and actually managed to find help this way; a local secondary school sends student volunteers to help at our twins club – there are many ways of finding help but obviously these completely depend on where you live.

I went on recruitment walks

When Jess and Isla were first born and looked so sweet, innocent and mostly asleep in the double buggy, I went out for what I jokingly called recruitment walks to collect telephone numbers of neighbouring ladies, their grand-daughters and other seemingly trustworthy people. I never intended to leave my babies alone with them; I just thought it would be good to have someone to call on when things got a bit hectic, or to entertain the babies whilst I was cooking dinner etc.

On one occasion, after a pretty rough night, I just wasn't in the mood for chatting to people and displaying myself as the proud twin mum of three, pushing my funky big double buggy loaded to the brim with my beautiful entourage of little children – I just wanted

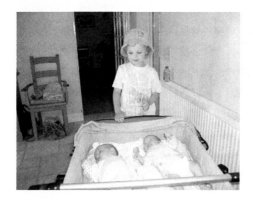

All loaded up and ready for another 'recruitment walk'.

to be grumpy and for those little four months old screamers to go to sleep, when a lady I hardly knew forced her number upon me. I didn't ring her until the winter when the girls were ten months old and we had yet another lunchtime drama during half term break and all my teenage helpers had gone skiing. I found myself in the kitchen with three ill, hungry and overtired children dangling off my legs and arms and little hope of preparing any food when my eyes caught sight of that little piece of paper she'd given me half a year ago. I rang her, she came over straight away, helped warm up some food and cuddled a screaming Isla. The funny thing was that she really seemed to enjoy her-self despite all the crying and the chaos in the house. She was so pleased that I had phoned her and had given her the opportunity to help. Before she left, she quickly reloaded the dishwasher and believe it or not, the dishwasher really cleaned the dishes even though she didn't put the plates in the "correct" place.

People want to help and you could even go as far as to say that letting them help you is helping them by giving them the opportunity to make a difference. Remember that people, in general, love babies, but they adore twins!

I treated myself to a cleaner for the first weeks

Many books recommend getting a cleaner for the first few months and I think it's great advice if you can afford it. Fairy-Mary came in twice a week, one hour on Tuesdays and 1.5 hours on Fridays, she vacuumed, cleaned the bathrooms and maintained a comforting level of tidiness in the house. Bliss! We arranged everything with her whilst I was pregnant; she started a short while before the birth as the last weeks of pregnancy weren't great for vacuuming or scrubbing the loo. But we were also absolutely fine without a cleaner, we just lowered our expectations. It was a sweet luxury for a while.

Hiring a cleaner, nanny, babysitter serves the purpose to reduce stress, but it can be stressful if you don't outline your expectations.

When hiring someone, outline exactly what you expect of them, if possible, put it in writing. When hiring a cleaner, for example, try and create a brief cleaning plan (can be scribbled down on any kind of paper using crayons or whatever else comes to hand), what rooms, what you want them to do. Not an hour of dusting in the spare room but actually clean the floors and the toilets instead. If you have a nanny ask to tidy up any toys before they leave, outline what older siblings are not allowed to do and what household jobs they can do when the babies are asleep. If you write it down it will be easier for them to follow and you don't have the stress of having to remind them, repeating yourself or even falling out over it.

How to avoid disappointment

Unpaid help is great as it's mostly from people who enjoy spending time with you and your children and who don't have a financial interest. It's great not having to pay, especially when you're not intending to leave the helper alone with the babies. The downside of unpaid help, even if it's from friends and family, is that it can be less reliable and sometimes a helper being late or not turning up at all is just the last thing you need. There were a couple of times when my first volunteer was supposed to be coming for three hours in the afternoon, and I found myself looking forward to it so much that the

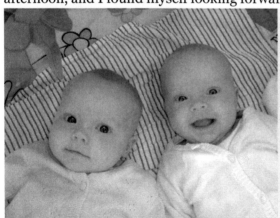

Ella and Amilia enjoying a bit of entertainment.

disappointment of her not showing up was worse than not having any help in the first place.

On one occasion I would have taken my five months old very unhappy twins for a walk at 12:55 but thought I'd just hang on in there for another five minutes until my volunteer was due to arrive. At 13:30 she still hadn't arrived and when I phoned her, I quickly realised that she'd simply forgotten and I was close to tears. I was upset with her and with myself for waiting for her arrival and with my babies for crying so much and I was really stressed. And I decided to eliminate these situations in the future and worked out a plan to avoid unnecessary stress and disappointment:

- If someone plans to come and visit, tell them where they can find you if you're not at home. For example, a usual route you take with the buggy, they could walk towards you. You shouldn't think there would be the need to in the age of mobile communication but you might just want to get walking in your slippers and have no idea where your mobile phone currently resides.

- Ask your visitors to cancel early or warn of delays early.

- Accept that the novelty of twin babies will wear off and helpers might go through phases where they will be less

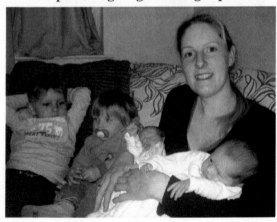

My sister and her helping hands.

available to help you, your younger helpers for example might be unavailable during revision for exams. Don't ever take it personally when they aren't around as much as they used to be, it's totally normal and will probably change again.

A few twin mum quotes

"I coped well in the first year and refused offers of help. Then when things started getting tough, I felt like I couldn't ask people for help. I wish I had – it would have made life so much easier!"
Sarah, mum to Jess and Lily

"Come, visit and tidy my house, just let me take a break and cuddle my babies."
Suzie, mum to Poppy, Joel, Orla and Lily

"My biggest struggle was to get my first born to pre-school on time even though it was just a short walk from our house. I was really lucky that other mums offered to help and were happy to walk past our house in the morning to collect him."
Christine, mum to Ben, Inca and Lenny

"My home start volunteer was an absolute life saver."
Julie, mum to Holly, Harrison and Daniel

Glimpse into
the future

A little pool side story - Jess and Isla are six months old and on Wednesdays you find us at the local pool for Jacob's swim-ming lessons and believe it or not there are actually three other mums of twins and they all happen to be identical, what are the chances? Anyway, it's a bit like an underground unofficial twins club and every topic under the sun is being discussed whilst our offspring learn to stand the 'waves' at the leisure centre pool. Angela has the most gripping stories to tell. Her totally adorable daughters must have been far from adorable when they were babies. One thing she said really made me think: "The hardest thing was to admit that I needed help and that no matter how super organised a person I always used to be, I couldn't do it on my own and it doesn't make me a less good mother." Mums want the best for their children and we all strive to be the best mum we can be. During pregnancy I even looked forward to the challenge of having two babies and doing it all on my own. I thought with the right organisation and preparation I could do it alone and be the shining super mum, who at the end of the day could say she coped very well all by herself. Now the girls are six months old and reality looks very different. Tonight I am feeling extremely proud of myself for all the help I organised, I have seen so many different people today, had a nice cup of tea and I had a shower! How great am I?

Jess and Isla are now 19 months old, Jacob has started school and life is just so much easier now! The girls are now walking and much happier, they have learned the art of eating and the weaning mess has come to an end. They eat exactly the same as we do; they feed themselves and play happily alongside one another, as long as I keep play interesting for them. I no longer feel I could do with help in the mornings or at dinner time, unless they are really unwell or overtired, but I have learned to avoid these situations. If one of them makes a fuss and hangs on my leg whilst I get dinner ready, I just place her in the travel cot (or as we call it the trouble cot) in the playroom, with some toys, and just carry on preparing dinner.

They understand so much now and get very excited when I tell them to get their shoes and coats as we are about to leave the house to get big brother Jacob from school. I still ask for help if I want to go somewhere like an indoor play centre as it's just more fun to be able to concentrate on one of them. When we go for a walk, I get Jacob to hold Jess's or Isla's hand, which is very cute and works a treat. All three children sleep in the same bedroom now and it's even become easy putting them to bed by myself. Dinner at 4:30, bath at 5:30, cereal, milk from a beaker at 6:00, brush teeth, upstairs for a play and last run around, 6:35 kiss, cuddle, bed and I head back downstairs and have a cup of tea.

Jess and Isla have just turned three. Where have those babies gone? Life is still busy and it's still great to have help now and then, but ever since the girls started to understand the concept of consequences, life suddenly got much easier. When we go food shopping, I have a chat with them in the car park explaining what I expect of them once we leave the car. This for example includes holding my hand in the car park and to be kind to one another in the supermarket. I also tell them what we are not going to buy. The consequence of them sticking to the rules is normally that they are allowed to sit in the funny music bus by the checkout and have a little treat whilst I pay. They are old enough now to go to swimming classes without me having to get in the water and they are so excited and happy to be doing it all by themselves - with one another of course. It's absolutely lovely to take them out now.

Older Siblings

As mentioned before, Jacob had just turned three when his twin sisters were born. He did incredibly well. During the last leg of the pregnancy he was getting quite frus-trated with having a mum who had turned into a complete non-mover. He was quite upset that I was no longer allowed to carry him around, cuddling up on my lap didn't really work either and he kept asking me:

"When will they come out so you can carry me again?".

During this time I really appreciated anyone entertaining Jacob; I was tired and my legs were swollen and I welcomed all offers by friends and family to take Jacob out so I could sleep or just rest. Once the babies were born I had my hands full with them, and luckily the offers to take Jacob out kept coming but it didn't take long until I realised that I would actually prefer if people wouldn't take him out but just stick around and keep an eye on the girls so I could spend some quality time with Jacob. So when Granny came over or when my Home Start volunteer came around, I would always try and give Jacob some undivided attention, even if just for half an hour.

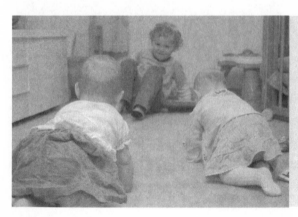

There is nowhere to hide from the nosy twin sisters.

{CHAPTER 2}

SUPPORT AND SOCIALISING

It's incredibly liberating and powerful to talk to other mothers:
Realising that you are not alone, that you are doing the right
thing and that your thoughts are completely normal.

I suppose all mums with little children agree: you've got to get out and meet other people in order to stay balanced and happy and to find support with the various challenges and changes that come with having children. When I had Jacob I went to the weekly breastfeeding café, swimming lessons, baby gym, baby clinic, baby massage, mother and toddler group, shopping in town and many trips to the playground. With two babies it's slightly different as for most of the activities listed above you would be better off bringing a helper along. The trick with twins is to choose suitable activities and places and to be well prepared.

Some days I felt exhausted or worried and whenever I needed to talk, I found that other mums were just the best source of support. Friends without children didn't quite understand what all the fuss was about, but they were great when it came to distracting and cheering me up and they actually made me realise there still was a world out there away from nappies and Postman Pat. Talking to other mums was what kept me going; simply knowing that you are not alone is such a powerful tool.

I interviewed Theresa for this book, she is a mental health nurse and she told me that peer support is widely acknowledged as the most successful form of postnatal support.

Theresa says "In most cases mums don't need to see mental health professionals, they need to go and see other mums to understand that what they are feeling and thinking is totally normal". And if you ask me, the most suitable place there could possibly be to find support is your local twins and multiples club.

THE LOCAL TWINS CLUB: EVERY TWIN MUM'S SAFE HAVEN!

If there is a Twins and Multiples Club where you are: Go! This is the one place where you will feel normal and understood, where you see parents with older twins that have been where you are now, who can offer you support, advice, a hug or just simply are the living proof that you can do it and that things will get easier when your babies get older.

I remember my first visit to my local Twins and Multiples Club, I was 24 weeks pregnant. I walked through the door and felt like I was entering a whole new world – 'twinland'. I couldn't help but feel amazed by all those lovely twin babies and twin toddlers. I felt so privileged to soon be part of the exclusive club and at the same time anxious.

I went whilst I was pregnant as I wanted to talk to fellow twin

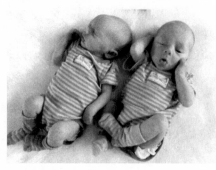

Hattie and Bea, part of the gang at my local Twins and Multiples Club.

mums where the twins had also shared the placenta. I wanted to find out if anyone had given birth naturally as I really didn't like the idea of having a c-section. I wasn't sure how it would affect my ability to breastfeed and look after my three year old son. I spoke to Sarah, who later became a great friend; she had had a c-section and breastfed without any problems. This sounded very promising.

Two years later I became chair of my local Twins and Multiples Club and I loved giving back what the club gave me when I needed it the most. I recommend any expectant twin parent to visit their local club during pregnancy as it's a brilliant way of getting an idea of what lies ahead. It provides the opportunity to collect telephone numbers for the last leg of the pregnancy when you just need to talk to someone who can confirm that you will be able to last another week or two and that those swollen hands and feet will vanish once the babies have arrived .

You won't find any of the competition you find between singleton mums, especially first time mums. Here it doesn't matter who walks first, talks first – all that matters is that your twins are here and that you are now a resident of twinland. It's also a great place to pick up second hand equipment and test double buggies, discuss sources for help, find other suitable groups and activities and much more. Tuesday mornings are a fixture in my life – one of us would have to be really ill for us to miss Twins Club. Visit www.tamba.org.uk to find a UK Club, try www.nomotc.org for the US, www.amba.org.au for Australia and www.multiplebirthscanada.org for Canada.

"This is the only place where I don't feel like a freak but a normal parent surrounded by other normal parents."
Chloe, mum to Hector and Felix

GENERAL BABY AND TODDLER GROUPS

I found that groups designed for first time singleton mums weren't that suitable. I walked in with my two babies and conversations stopped. Whatever problems these ladies had just been debating – I had them twice – or maybe their worries had just magically disappeared and been replaced with sheer delight that they only had one baby to cuddle, carry, change and feed. I found myself answering the same questions over and over again. And no one had a hand free to give me a hand when I needed it. So I didn't really bother with the 'normal' baby clinic. Groups where toddlers were welcome turned out to be much more suitable as there were mums with more than one child and their lives were similar.

Sometimes mothers would tell me they'd had their children so close together "It was just like having twins!" and I couldn't help but think "Well, lucky you, you managed to have a shag half way through giving birth!" Once the novelty of twins had worn off and everyone knew I had twins, we actually moved on to things we really had in common due to the fact that we had more than

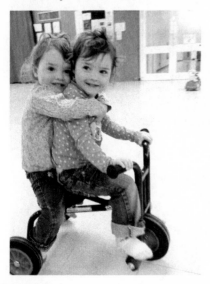

*Isla and Jess
are having fun
at the toddler
group.*

one child and that was great. Just the general understanding that you have more than one to look after, that you might ask to look after one whilst you go and change the other one's nappy is great.

HOSPITAL GROUPS

Many hospitals with neonatal care wards offer support groups and meetings for families with premature children. It's worthwhile asking the hospital or other twin mums to see what's available.

"I felt totally out of place when going to ordinary toddler groups as my twins were so tiny and fragile and I was scared what they might catch. I only ever went to my hospitals neonatal group as all parents there were in the same boat and wouldn't come along if their children were unwell."

Anonymous

BREASTFEEDING GROUPS

To find a local breastfeeding group ask at your hospital, your Children's Centre, your midwife or your health professional.

La Leche League for example is an international, non-profit, non-sectarian organisation dedicated to providing education, information, support, and encouragement to women wanting to breastfeed. Their website and booklets are very helpful. Their website can be found under www.laleche.org

LOCAL CHURCH, CHAPEL OR OTHER PLACE OF WORSHIP

I found this a good place to find help and support alike. I am not talking about sitting in a cold stone building here, trying to keep two babies quiet during a one hour church service and putting a three year old Spiderman on a lead. I chose coffee mornings, play mornings and family services with Sunday school instead. I am not suggesting you convert to any belief – my atheist friends enjoyed the church toddler groups just as much as I did.

The people I met through church were so practical; the most amazing thing was that during the three weeks after coming home from hospital they cooked dinners for us! I couldn't believe it when the first person turned up on our doorstep, 5pm with a home cooked beef stew complete with dumplings and pudding. Wow! And every evening someone else showed up with a home made curry or pasta bake, one Sunday evening we even had a full English roast dinner!

So, it's all about choosing the right activities and places. Let me tell you about:

THE ART OF GETTING TWO BABIES OUT THE CAR, BUS OR TRAIN AND INTO A BUILDING

• Take your double buggy, check the location is accessible with your buggy and there is space to park it.

• Use a double carrier; however they can be quite a strain on your back. Getting two babies out of car seats and into a double front carrier can be fiddly. I practised at home on my bed. It only works for a few months when the babies are at the right size and age and gets you a huge amount of attention should you fancy some.

• Use a front and back carrier or two slings at the same time, this is easier and works much longer and probably works out cheaper. Still quite heavy but looks very cute and also allows you to hold a siblings hand.

• Have one in a sling or carrier and the other one in a car seat or on your hip.

• Have one in a sling or carrier and the other in a single buggy.

• Ask for a helper to meet you at the car and take one baby each.

• When they get older you could try a single buggy with a buggy board.

• Once they can walk you could try letting one walk whilst the other is in the buggy, sling, carrier.

• Walk holding both their hands and hope that no-one has a melt down or walk with them using (double) reins.

Once my girls could stand, I soon realised that there was this brief moment of danger when you take the second one out the car seat whilst number one is already stood waiting next to the car. I taught them very early to stand right next to me, not to move, hold on to my leg or sit down when possible so I could safely take my eyes off them for a moment to unload their twin. Once they were capable of climbing out of their car seats I started to unbuckle them from inside the car and then they would climb over to one and the same side and leave the car on that side. Teaching them to safely climb in and out their car seats is also going to be appreciated by your back.

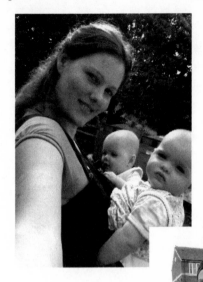

*Twin baby
carrier*

*Two single
baby carriers*

*Two baby
slings*

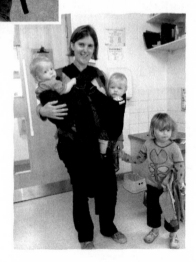

THE ART OF NAPPY CHANGING ON THE GO

Some singleton mums turn nappy changing into an art form, they steer their beautiful small buggy into the change room, have a play with their baby, carefully and slowly change the nappy, wipe and cream the little bottom, place everything neatly back into the cute little changing bag, have another cuddle and play and leave the facilities around ten minutes later with a gracious smile on their face.

I am entitled to say this as I was a singleton mum once and nappy changing was far from being a stressful experience. With two babies I quickly realised that most changing facilities, especially those in parks and the city centre are just not designed for double buggies. You don't really want to leave one of them outside to guard the buggy, so in you go carrying both. If they can stand and are willing to stand a little while then you're lucky as toilet floors tend to be too disgusting to sit one baby on the floor whilst you change the other.

Mine didn't want to stand around, so I became an absolute pro in the art of nappy changing on my lap. Once, whilst on holiday, I did a 45 second poo-nappy lap change aboard an open side bus, taking us at a considerable speed through a pack of monkeys at a Spanish wildlife park. Basically what you do is, you sit down with your legs pushed together, you cover your upper thighs with a flannel or a fresh nappy and then you lay your baby sideways or bum facing you on your home made changing mat and hold your baby with one hand whilst the other hand does the job. This takes a bit of practice, as of course the aim is to change the nappy without dropping the baby or staining yourself.

I practised at home and it really didn't take long at all. This way I could completely avoid having to leave my buggy at all. The buggy also provided excellent cover when in a busy place. Later on

I moved on to standing up nappy changing or sitting down nappy changing where I would place the fresh nappy on my knee, the girls would sit down onto the nappy and I could do it up quite easily.

THINGS YOU SHOULD ALWAYS HAVE IN YOUR CAR OR UNDER YOUR BUGGY

There is nothing more annoying then having to go home despite having a good time, just because of toilet accidents and spillages. So here are some ideas for items to permanently leave in the car or under the buggy, without the need to pack them or the danger to forget them:

- Spare nappies, maybe even a size up so they don't outgrow them should you not need them for a while. You can fold the top of the nappy over to make them fit, I had to do this all the time when Isla was first born as even the premature baby nappies were too big for her.

- Spare clothes, again maybe a size up, you could buy them second hand so it's not a problem if you forget about them and end up never using them.

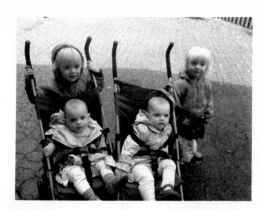

Twins Jess and Lily pushing their little twin friends Jess and Isla whilst mums Sarah and Kerri socialise.

- Hand towels and plastic carrier bags to clean up and conceal any unwanted surprises.

- Emergency snacks and water.

IT'S YOUR LIFE AND YOUR TIME, SPEND IT THE WAY YOU WANT

On a holiday in Florida, when I was 20, I started chatting to a tour guide who had spent five years living with the Hopi, a tribe of Native Americans living in a reservation in Arizona. Some translate Hopi into "Peaceful people", and I enjoyed hearing about their traditions and ceremonies and I really liked one of their mottos which was something along the lines of: "The greatest gift you can give someone, is the time you spend with them as time is the one thing you really only have a limited supply of." How true!

And it's when you have little children, then you really start to notice the shortage of time and you suddenly no longer want to spend time doing things you don't enjoy (unless they are necessary). Of course, sometimes the events we dread the most turn out to be the most fun. But sometimes you wish you had declined in the first place. So, don't go to that pretentious birthday meal you're not going to enjoy. It's your time, your life! And you now have two or more perfect reasons to say "no, thanks".

SUPPORT WITHOUT HAVING TO LEAVE THE HOUSE

There are times when getting out of the house to socialise is simply not possible. I spent several weeks house bound as Jess and Isla just seemed to pick up every bug under the sun. I felt stuck at home and desperate to talk to other mums. Luckily there are various sources of support you can use without having to leave the house, numbers you can call when you feel down and things to read to make you feel better. Here are some sources I found helpful:

Twins and Multiple Births Association TAMBA (UK)
I mention TAMBA various times throughout this book and I recommend joining to any twin parent. Let me quote them to explain what they are all about: "TAMBA is a UK charity set up by parents of twins, triplets and higher multiples and interested professionals. Our campaigns, research and support services directly help thousands of parents and professionals meet the unique challenges that multiple birth families face."

I joined the day I found out I was expecting twins and I visited the website on a daily basis whilst I was pregnant and I found so much support during the worrying times of the pregnancy. My biggest worry was Isla's poor growth. How small would she be? Would she be OK? I posted my concerns on the forum, which is a great place to talk to people who have either experienced what you are feeling, thinking or worrying about or they might just be in the same boat at the same time. The replies I received were amazing; one mum sent me pictures of her teeny tiny premature babies just after birth and the same twins on their second birthday. Those pictures really kept me going.

TAMBA offers helpful publications and videos which are all free to download for members. Tamba run antenatal and preparing for parenthood courses, I am one of their facilitators for the preparing for parenthood classes. These courses are excellent and I wish I had been able to attend one myself. You will need to leave the house in order to attend these courses but as you do this whilst you are pregnant they might offer a good opportunity to meet and stay in touch with local parents of multiples. Tamba offers a free phone listening service on 0800 138 0509. Open every day between 10am and 1pm and between 7pm and 10pm or you can email asktwinline@tamba.org.uk. Website: www.tamba.org.uk or search for TAMBA on Facebook.

The National Organization of Mothers of Twins Clubs, Inc NOMOTC (USA)

NOMOTC is a non-profit organisation based in the USA. Their work is dedicated to supporting families of multiple birth children through education, research, and networking, in partnering with local support groups, health care providers, researchers, and educators. Their aim is to aid parents of multiples and to raise public awareness of the unique qualities of multiple birth families. Website: www.nomotc. org, Facebook: www.facebook.com/NOMOTC

Australian Multiple Birth Association AMBA

AMBA was formed in 1974; they are the only national support organisation for multiple-birth families and individuals in Australia. AMBA's mission is to function as an effective network to support multiple birth families. "We fulfil our mission by providing support, education, research, and advocacy both nationally and internationally to individuals, families, member clubs, and organisations that have a personal or professional interest in multiple birth issues." Their website is www.amba.org.au, Facebook: ww.facebook.com/ AustralianMultipleBirthAssociation

Bliss www.bliss.org.uk

Bliss is the UK charity working to provide the best possible care and support for all premature and sick babies and their families. The website and their booklets are an invaluable source for info about neonatal care and equipment used, tube feeding, breastfeeding, kangaroo care, coming home, development and so much more. Some booklets are handed out in hospital but it's better not to rely on it and download them beforehand. The Bliss booklet about expressing and breastfeeding was my bible when I was in hospital.

The Bliss free help and advice line 0500 618140 is open Monday to Friday 9am to 9pm, you can also email them: hello@bliss.org.uk.

CRY-SIS www.cry-sis.org.uk

Cry-sis is a well respected UK charity offering support for families with excessively crying, sleepless and demanding babies. They have developed a checklist on what to do when baby is crying, they kindly agreed to let me include it in this book, you can find the checklist in the third chapter. The Cry-sis telephone helpline 08451 228669 is available every day of the year between 9.00am and 10.00pm. Callers are referred to a trained volunteer member of Cry-sis who has had personal experience of crying or sleep problems within their own family.

General Parenting Books

Books are a great source for support and advice but one thing to remember is that it isn't always right just because it's published in a book (says she writing a book).

There are many 'Baby Trainer' books out there and with them there is a lot of controversy over how much you should attempt to 'train' a baby. I believe any book you read should help and support you, if it stresses you out – chuck it in the bin and read something else. I mention books I found helpful throughout this book and I have a book section with order links on my website www.lifewithtwins.co.uk.

If I could start all over again, I would have read the following books much earlier:

- **What Every Parent Needs To Know** by Margot Sunderland (I think every parent should be given a free copy of this book when they have their first baby), Publisher: Dorling Kindersley

- **The Wonder Weeks** by Frans Plooij Ph.D and Hetty van de Rijt Ph.D, Publisher: Kiddy World Promotions B.V.

- **Toddler Taming** by Dr. Christopher Green, Publisher: Vermilion

- **Practical Parenting: Sleep** by Siobhan Stirling, Publisher: Hamlyn

- **Mothering Multiples: Breastfeeding and Caring for Twins or More** by La Leche League, Karen Kerkhoff Gromada, Publisher: Overseas Editions New

Facebook and other networks

Like many other clubs across the globe, we set up a private, closed Facebook group for our local Twins and Multiples Club and all sorts of questions are being asked and answered via computer, laptop, tablet or phone. We share stories, photographs and check up on one another. Some of the group members have never actually made it to our real life group meetings, yet the page seems a helpful place to find support.

I remember some days I was really exhausted and just wanted to be alone and not answer any text messages, yet a little piece of paper in my pocket told me to "share my thoughts and feelings with at least one person each day" and the A4 sheet on my front door told me to "get out the door and start walking". I obeyed my own rules and soon started to feel better. Please feel free to copy the next page.

For your front door

> # *Life is out there!*
>
> # *Get out and*
>
> # *start walking!*

For your pocket/wallet

Talk to a friend
or family member
each and every day!
Especially when you don't
feel like talking.

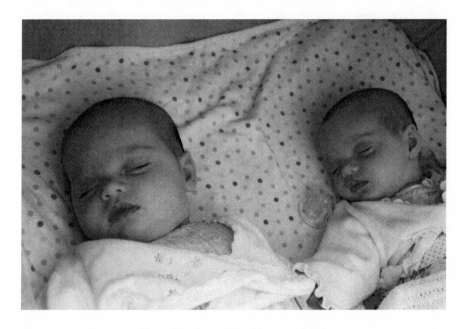

Sleeping beauties Jess and Isla.

{CHAPTER 3}

SLEEP

"If only I could give depressed women sleep,
I could cure so many of them!"
Theresa, Mental Health Nurse

Isn't it funny how our relationship to sleep changes throughout life? As small children we try to avoid going to bed at all costs, as teenagers many don't even leave their beds before noon, as young adults we live for the moment and have an "I can sleep when I am dead" attitude – we don't really pay much respect to sleep before we have children. But now as parents with little babies sleep has become a rare and precious gift, we spend hours thinking and talking about sleep, sleep is of such importance – only problem is that we're just not getting enough of it!

Lack of sleep is a common side effect of having babies or small children and one thing I found to be of major importance was to understand the effect lack of sleep was having on my ability to cope even with the smallest of tasks, the effect on feelings towards my children and my general well being!

The development babies and toddlers go through during the first years of their lives is simply incredible! (Read more details about their development in the fourth chapter.) So many "firsts", so much to learn and take in and they have to process it all whilst they sleep. An adult would already struggle to sleep if they had to move house or start a new job, a baby might learn to walk or suddenly feel fear of someone leaving the room and never returning – and they are expected to go to bed and sleep through the night. That might not happen. Chances are your babies will sleep well one month and not so well the next, they pick up bugs, have nightmares or simply wake up wanting a cuddle. Circumstances change all the time and it's an ongoing process of creating positive sleep associations and at the same time creating trust.

Some weeks were challenging and I found myself thinking that I had failed completely. Looking back I realise I hadn't failed at all, as the sleepless nights were just as much part of teaching my children how to sleep well, as those nights when they peacefully slept through. I believe it was during those difficult times, when they just wanted to be with me and be rocked back to sleep, that they learned that they can trust me to be there for them and that they could feel safe in their beds and bedrooms. But this also makes for very tired parents. You simply don't realise just how tired you can get until you have your first baby and even more so with two babies. But it doesn't last forever! I promise.

The only real cure for lack of sleep is SLEEP! Common advice is to sleep when baby sleeps; with twins it just isn't that easy. But there are many ideas on how to try and get more sleep and ideas on how to cope with little sleep.

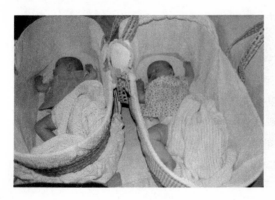

Isla and Jess taking a daytime nap in their separate Moses baskets.

"Me sleep – you love me."
Maya 30 months

SLEEP FOR THE BABIES

For many parents the first time they ever think about their babies' sleep is when they work out where their babies will actually be sleeping, not how. And it's whilst making these sleep arrangements that many of us first come across Sudden Infant Death Syndrome (SIDS). I didn't even want to think about this topic when I was pregnant, as it scared me so much. But it's very important to know about SIDS in order to make a conscious, informed decision about where your babies will be sleeping. The cause of SIDS is still unexplained but there has been a lot of research which has led to recommendations on how to reduce the risk. I have taken the following recommendations from The Lullaby Trust and added further info where appropriate:

• Always place your baby on their back to sleep. (This simple recommendation has reduced cot death rates by 50% since 1994.)

• Keep your baby smoke free during pregnancy and after birth.

• Place your babies to sleep in a separate cot or individual Moses basket in the same room as you for the first six months. (Research has found no increased risk for twins sharing a cot; they should however NOT share a Moses basket.)

• Breastfeed your baby, if you can. (The German Study of Sudden Infant Death found that breastfeeding reduced the risk of SIDS by 50% at all ages throughout infancy. The researchers suggest including the advice to breastfeed through six months of age in SIDS recommendations.)

• Use a firm, flat, waterproof mattress in good condition.

• Never sleep on a sofa or in an armchair with your baby.

• Don't sleep in the same bed as your baby if you smoke, drink or take drugs or are extremely tired, if your baby was born prematurely or was of low birth-weight.

• Avoid letting your baby get too hot.

• Don't cover your baby's face or head while sleeping or use loose bedding.

• Place your baby on their back in the 'feet to foot' position. This is where the baby's feet are placed at the foot of the cot, so they can't wriggle down under any blankets.

I followed the above advice and always felt that what I was doing was safe. Jacob moved into his own bedroom when he was nine months old, up till then we used a bed side cot and once I finished breastfeeding I would just move him over into the bed side cot. With two babies the logistics suddenly changed. In the beginning they slept in separate Moses baskets which stood next to me on the vacant mattress in our double guest bed, pushed against the wall so they couldn't fall off.

Once they outgrew the baskets, they moved into their own cots in our bedroom. When they were nine months old they moved into their own bedroom, but I would still let them sleep next to me if they were ill or just wouldn't settle; they were always on the adjacent mattress and I was never under the influence of anything other than the wish for everyone to sleep. I was tired, but there was never any danger of me rolling onto them or of them falling out of bed – and we all slept.

So all was good and I was happily writing the following pages of this book when Professor R G Carpenter published his latest findings on 20.May 2013 and I had to rethink whether I could actually go ahead and publish this book in its current form as it does mention bed sharing. Carpenter's conclusion is: "Bed sharing for sleep when the parents do not smoke or take alcohol or drugs increases the risk of SIDS. Risks associated with bed sharing are greatly increased when combined with parental smoking, maternal alcohol consumption and/or drug use. A substantial reduction of SIDS rates could be achieved if parents avoided bed sharing."

Many professionals criticise that the study is missing vital points, for example it doesn't consider whether bed sharing was planned (versus unplanned) or whether the parents were aware of SIDS.

Educating parents on how to safely sleep near their babies is important and the message to all my readers is:

Please visit www.lullabytrust.org.uk or the website of the American SIDS Institute www.sids. org and read up on cot death, be sensible and make an informed decision about your sleeping arrangements.

The Lullaby Trust has kindly granted permission for me to include their easy reading cards in this book. For a downloadable version of these, please visit www.lullabytrust.org.uk.

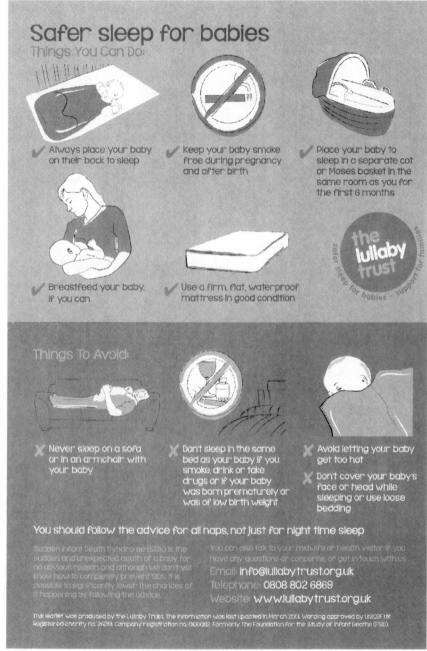

How to get your children to sleep

Getting our children to sleep at night is one of the biggest talking points in raising children, us professionals (parents) spend days and nights discussing strategies, successes and downfalls. We know exactly for how long Molly and Ellie slept last night, what time Thomas woke up and when Sophie went down, how little sleep all their parents have had and how much coffee or tea they'll need in order to make it through the day.

The single most important piece of advice I was ever told when it comes to sleep: Put your baby to bed BEFORE she falls asleep!

If you can get your baby to LOVE and TRUST the place where she sleeps – then you're on to a winner! It's all about creating positive sleep associations and this can take some time and may require a great deal of patience. I have collected some popular advice on how to improve babies sleep:

- Establish a daytime routine for sleeping and feeding.

- Make sure they don't have too much / or too little daytime sleep. Overtired children don't sleep well either – search for "baby sleep" on the NHS website www.nhs.org for more info.

- Make sure they take in enough food throughout the day. Visit the NHS or World Health Organisation www.who.int for more information.

- Establish a bedtime routine / ritual.

- Fresh air in the daytime makes for better sleep at night.

- Sing familiar lullabies at bedtime.

- Dim the lights and keep noise down when preparing for bed.

- Put them to bed awake, if they fall asleep during a feed, try and arouse them a little so they know they are now in bed and no longer in your arms.

• Have a good night phrase, repeat whenever you put them to bed.

• Don't change anything in the room once you have left.

• Make the change from many naps, to two naps, then down to one day-time nap and eventually to no daytime sleep when the time has come to do so. (Again, search for "baby sleep" on the NHS website for up to date guidelines.)

• If they use a dummy, leave plenty of dummies in their cot so they can easily locate one by themselves rather than you having to crawl under the cot at 3am. NEVER use a dummy with neckcord!

• Some babies like to be swaddled and the nurses in hospital trained me on how to safely swaddle my girls. Modern swaddling is nothing like what they used to do to babies hundreds of years ago when limbs and hips were damaged. For a while it was suggested that correct swaddling reduces the risk of SIDS, recent research now suggests a possible link between swaddling and SIDS. Guidelines keep changing all the time , so please ask health professionals and read up for yourself on www.nct.org. uk.

• Use a musical toy, for example one with a gentle glow, which you carry with you and switch on whenever it's time for a sleep. Seahorses seem to be a popular choice.

• If they wake up for a feed and they are entitled to one – easy! Chances are they just fall asleep once fed. Ideally you don't want to wake them when you change their nappy after the feed. Here are some ideas how to tackle it:

• Purely functional nappy changing with only very little light and no talking.

• Many mums and dads actually change the nappy half way through the feed to avoid waking baby when stuffed, happy and asleep.

• Some avoid wet wipes in the middle of the night and just replace a wet nappy. This obviously doesn't work with soiled nappies!

• Once the babies get a bit bigger some parents use nappies one size up to make them last longer. (You will need to fold over the top of the nappies to make them fit.)

During our stay in neonatal care the nurses used to dim the lights in the evening and reduce noise, setting the scene for bedtime.

We have a bed time routine which we established quite early on when the girls where a couple of months old. It's basically a bath, story, milk and bed – rhythm. I never would have thought I'd bath my children every night, and I didn't with my first born but the benefits of doing so are worth it, it doesn't have to be a proper bath anyway. Most nights we only fill the bath tub a bit so that the children can have a little splash around. It's more about the message that soon they'll be put to bed rather than anything else.

When it was time to go to sleep, we used to try and let them go to sleep in their own cots, without rocking or feeding them to sleep. When they were really little this didn't always happen as they would simply fall asleep after their milk feed. When they got a bit older I would always try and put them to bed awake and it did the trick with Jess, she just loves going to bed (most nights), she puts her arms up next to her head, she even smiles at me when I leave the room and then she just falls asleep. Isla is a different story. Because of her low birth weight in connection with all the worries about her during the pregnancy, I just couldn't help but cuddle her to sleep during the first months. I just couldn't let go and it was so lovely. I absolutely love the feeling when you cuddle your child to sleep, when they snuggle right into your neck and then you can feel their little warm body getting all relaxed and soft and you can feel how they drift off to sleep, all happy and pro-tected. It's wonderful! But it can be quite exhausting when this is the only way your child can go to sleep as evenings in my life are a very precious three hour window of time with my husband, cook dinner, get on the computer, watch a film or sit in our hot tub. (Yes, we have a hot tub in our little rear garden and it's the best purchase we have ever made!)

I normally was the one putting the girls to bed. I used to stick around a bit and make some gentle noises to let them know I was still there and they'd go to sleep. Sometimes that wasn't enough, and I have spent an awful lot of time pretending to be asleep on their bedroom floor only to crawl out on all fours once they have fallen asleep. Sometimes one of them was just too overtired, too upset about something or unwell and in that case I would just sit in the rocking chair for a couple of minutes with her and she'd either fall asleep in my arms or calm down enough to be put back and fall asleep in her cot. Sometimes I was just too knackered to stroke, sing, cuddle and pretend, plus the likelihood of falling asleep on the kid's bedroom floor was extremely high and the neck pain the morning after not that great. So sometimes when I knew that they were well and just

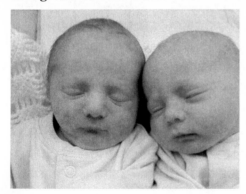

Oliver and Lewis giving mum Nicky a break.

crying because they were tired, I'd leave the room, take a deep breath and a couple minutes later I find them snoring their little heads off when I came back in to check on them. At times I found it really tough, I just wanted them to sleep and me to go downstairs, sit down and have some peace.

There was a time when they just wouldn't go down at all, they had both been ill and were teething. We spent all evening, every evening, trying to get them off to sleep. When Isla woke at night she would always want to be fed back to sleep but she'd wake up when I removed her from my breast - but I really couldn't sleep having her hard wired to my boob. Rocking, walking, cuddling, using a dummy, nothing worked, just constant breastfeeding. I was shattered. The nights were starting to cause real problems, I had milk blisters, we were all up, and no one was getting any sleep! Jess was up a lot too, they were probably waking one another we (naively) thought. But Jess wouldn't even go back to sleep when I fed her, she just wanted to be in my bed all night. I had tried signalling that the cot was a happy place all along, the room or the beds weren't an issue, it was just the fact that I wasn't there when she woke up at night.

So there we were discussing sleep training. We had to stop the nightly breastfeeding marathon and we had to get them to sleep in their own cots for at least the first part of the night. But how to? I didn't even know where to start with two babies, in one room? In separate rooms?

Did we have to sleep train them? On one hand I kept thinking: "They grow so quick and I love cuddling them, why not just cuddle them back to sleep and have them in my bed for a few years?" But when you have TWO babies in your bed, both wanting to sleep right next to you, you simply run into problems. The reality was that I wasn't getting any sleep, neither were Rich nor Jacob and they had to get up the next morning and go to work and to school.

I checked with my health visitor and she said they were old enough to drop night feeds. I phoned a parenting author who offers phone consultations and she suggested "controlled cry-ing". She came up with a plan, separate rooms, travel cots, leave them to cry, length of gaps between going in without talking or eye contact. We hadn't slept in what felt like ages, both girls were up all night, wanting attention. With our plan in hand we embarked on mission sleep training, it was a nightmare! Some nights I woke up in the middle of the night thinking "Where am I? Oh, the couch in the lounge. Any babies next to me? No – phew! Who is in the travel cot next door? Where's Rich? What time is it?" Such chaos: babies, toddlers and parents all over the place. I couldn't leave them to cry, it just goes against everything I believe in. If I left them for hours, surely all they'd learn is that mummy won't come when they cry. And I felt they would eventually pass out because they were exhausted, with stress levels running sky high.

They simply didn't understand that I was shattered and fed up because they would have happily spent all day with me, non stop cuddling me. But it's tough with two babies and sometimes leaving them to cry for a bit is unavoidable. An overtired child might just fall asleep within minutes, an overtired mum or dad could just take a deep breath and a break. Rich wanted to stick to the plan, I couldn't do it. We kept going back and forth. It certainly wasn't great for our relationship. We discussed a strategy in the daytime and I was determined to stick to it but then I threw it all overboard during the night and Rich wasn't impressed at all.

There is also the other end of the spectrum, the 'Continuum concept' the idea that a baby is still treated as part of the mother's body, you'd carry your baby all day and you'd co-sleep all night and as lovely as this might sound, it's not practical with two babies.

We settled somewhere in the middle and later found out that our chosen method is actually called "gradual withdrawal."

At bedtime I would stay in their room and fold some clothes, or leave the room and make some noise in the hallway just to let them know I was still there. If they cried we'd come back in and say: "shhhhhhh" and "mummy is just next door" and play some lullabies.

I did quit the night feeds and cuddled Isla for various nights, gave her water instead which she thought was outrageous; I stayed with her and tried to reassure her. Once she was over the milk-withdrawal I would keep her in her cot rather than cuddle her. Same for Jess, I kept her in her cot and reassured her. I tried to remind myself that their brain development is just incredible and there is so much to learn, understand and digest and most importantly that they don't stay little for ever. It took much longer than the three nights promised by cry it out and I was so tired but it felt right and fair.

When things settled down and the night feeds were a thing of the past, the girls always started the night in their own cots. They were one year old by now and we were starting to actually get some sleep. But once you've tasted sleep, you just want more and the thought of going back to sleepless nights was daunting. So when one woke towards the end of the night and a quick cuddle was just not enough to get her back to sleep – what options did I have? I could leave her to cry for a short while to see if she just fell asleep again but at the same time risk her waking her twin and her big brother, her

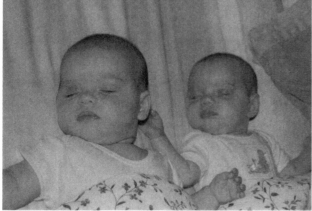

And they're finally asleep like babies (in my bed...).

dad and if we'd had direct neighbours then they'd be up too. Not a feasible option. Next option was to cuddle or rock her back to sleep and carefully transfer her back to bed, or to pretend to sleep on the floor next to her cot with my hand squeezed through the bars so I could hold her hand and then eventually crawl out the room on all fours avoiding the two squeaky floor boards. This was a plausible option but I would lose a huge amount of that much loved sleep so therefore wasn't always my most favoured choice. Last option was to take her back to my bed where she would instantly go back to sleep without waking her siblings and I would then get a sufficient amount of sleep – so for me this wasn't much of a personal choice whether to co sleep or not; for me it was simply the most effective way to get some sleep!

And yes sometimes they wake up knowing they might now be relocated to mummy's bed – and I can't even blame them be-cause I remember being a little girl and thinking of my parents bed as the safest place on the planet, completely monster-free and so warm. My sister must have felt the same as by sunrise she too was in our parent's big bed. But all my children do 360's in their sleep, they stick their fingers in my eyes, pull my hair and they snore. So as lovely as it all may sound to have them in my bed, it's really just to get a little more sleep towards the end of the night.

A quote from one of my favourite parenting books:

"Parents may wonder if their baby is crying to manipulate them, especially when they hear comments from well-meaning friends and family such as "Just leave him. He's just trying to control you. Give in now and you will suffer later." We now know its neurobiologically inaccurate. To manipulate an adult, a baby needs power of clear thought, and for that he needs a part of his brain thats not even established, this means he is not capable of thinking much about anything, let alone manipulating his parents."

From the book: What Every Parent Needs To Know by Margot Sunderland, Publisher: Dorling Kindersley

All parents are different!

I asked fellow twin mums about sleep training and sleep strategies and received a great range of answers, I think we all have to find something that works for our unique situation and our ever so unique babies. Please read below what other parents did:

"From as soon as we got home from hospital, we would bath
the boys at 6pm, not come downstairs, feed at 6:30pm
and place in cribs whether they were awake or had fallen
asleep during feeding. Even though I followed that routine
religiously only one twin would settle and sleep through
from 13 weeks old. The other one to this day is still a very
light sleeper and takes ages to settle."
Gillian, mum to Joshua and Oliver

"As soon as the twins came home we would put them to sleep
after their bottle. Basically they went down in their Moses
baskets (now cots) awake and would settle themselves to
sleep. They slept through the night from about 16 weeks
and to this day will sleep for about 12 hours, unless they
are poorly. When they were small and woke for feeds, I
would feed them and then put them straight back down.
I think whatever you do it is great to have a routine that
you stick to, so that your child can fully
understand what is happening. "
Zoe, mum to Ellis, Sophia and Ethan

"We still feed to sleep and then co-sleep at 16 months and it works for us. We started a loose bedtime routine at seven months and now they sleep 8pm-7.30am with a couple of wake ups each overnight. They have never been great sleepers but that's ok."
Rachael, mum to Harriet and Beatrice

"We got them into a routine early on. They slept through the night from ten weeks which is when we put them into their own rooms. They quite often fall asleep on their last bottle, but if not we put them in awake. We always put them in their cots awake in the day too."
Heidi, mum to Ellie and Brad

"We started a bedtime routine when Oliver and Jack were eight weeks old. We gave them a bottle at 6pm, followed by a bath and then put them to bed at 7pm. Oliver kept crying for no apparent reason and it wasn't really until they were 19 months that they started sleeping through the night. They are now two years old and frequently wake through the night."
Ingrid, mum to Oliver and Jack (At the time of publication Ingrid was expecting her second set of twins!)

"We just co-slept to get some sleep! I know this sounds crazy but honestly it meant I got sleep and sleep deprivation is

something I can't handle. I have found mine won't sleep in a cot but will in a travel cot - no idea why. The times I've been most stressed, were when I've been trying to follow books and advice. One thing my mother said was just do what you have to do to get some sleep - if I hadn't, I think I would have literally been a zombie." Tarryn, mum to Nathan and Joshua

"We did the bedtime routine from early on, fitting in with older brother. They slept together, in the same cot, until they were about six months old when they started to move around too much and disturb each other. They then had their own cots next to each other. They settled themselves to sleep and slept through after a late feed from about four months. They generally did the 7-7 sleep (and still need 12 hours at 4 1/2 years old). We found no real need to sleep train; they had each other for company and only woke when hungry. When one woke we woke the other and fed them together to avoid the constant feeding thing. They were both breast and bottle fed. They were much better sleepers and easier on that front than their singleton older brother!"

Tamsin, mum to Finley, Jake and Esme

"We got ours into a sleep routine as early as we could and they started going right through the night at three months. I breastfed them and at the beginning did this on demand, but when one of them woke in the night for a feed I would then always wake the other to feed and this worked for us, it quite quickly got them into the same sleep/feed pattern. Mine never co-slept at night (with each other or us) and were in separate Moses baskets and then separate cots. By 6/7 months old I would say our day and night routine was very structured with feeds and sleep and they were very in sync with each other, which was a blessing!"

Gemma, mum to Sophie and Heidi, Barrett

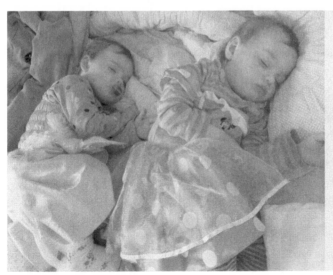

A couple of exhausted princesses.

Synchronised sleep

I really wanted the girls to sleep at the same time and tried the general advice of synchronising the whole day, especially the feeds. When one woke for a feed I would then wake the other in order to feed both, as I was breastfeeding this was a good plan as it took up less time to tandem feed. But if they woke and weren't due a feed but just awake I soon realised that the one woken up was really grumpy so I let her sleep longer and would open the curtains and let her wake up by herself.

I tried to get them to fall asleep at the same time though, either by placing them in their cots or by taking them for a walk or drive. They seemed to need different amounts of sleep, Isla the smaller one, slept a lot less than her sister. It was then that I realised how lovely it was when I had a quarter of an hour with just one of them.

I asked around how other twin mums get their twins to nap at the same time, here two of the replies:

"I take the boys for a drive and they will then fall asleep but they would wake when taken out of the car so I started napping in the car with them."
Hannah, mum to Charlie and Max

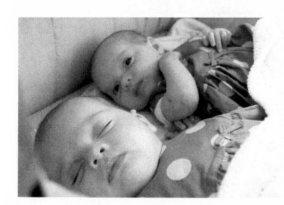

One awake,
one asleep.

"I have a strict routine, when it is naptime I put them to bed.
They stay there if they sleep or not."
Jennifer, mum to Sam and Sarah

When it all gets too much

There were a few nights, when all the love and understanding weren't able to overcome my desire and despair to sleep and I would start to feel irritated. That's when I woke my husband Rich, got him to take over regardless of him having to work the next morning as I had simply reached a point where I was no longer capable of doing it on my own.

Had I been a single mum I probably would have asked a friend or my mum to help me for a night or two. I met a twin mum who left her babies with her own mother for one night a week just to catch up on sleep that night. She says she couldn't have done it without that one night. But not all grandparents fancy taking on baby twins once a week.

It really helps to know how many hours of sleep are normal for a baby and how many naps they should have. I came across a book called "Sleep" by Siobhan Stirling which I personally found a really helpful and most importantly quick and easy read.

They say, too much sleep has been linked to a host of medical problems including diabetes, heart disease and increased risk of death. Lucky me, thanks to my children I should be safe.

SLEEP FOR YOU

During the first few months it wasn't a big deal to get up a lot at night, as I was breastfeeding on demand and had very, very low expectations of uninterrupted evenings and nights, I would just give them a feed and they would fall asleep during the feed. I didn't really get more than 90 minute chunks of sleep during the first three months and that was fine for me. Being little babies they spent a lot of time asleep, the first weeks they were only really up for a feed and then slept the rest of the time. I had plenty of opportunities to take naps too. Whilst in hospital I would take at least one daytime nap to make up for all the getting up at night. After a few months it got better, they were up less frequently at night and I got much faster at feeding and changing them at night and therefore managed to get a lot more night time sleep.

The girls are six months old whilst I am writing these pages. I go to bed much earlier than I used to, 10pm is a late night these days. Some evenings I feel ready to hit the pillows at 9pm but am torn between the wonderful idea of snuggling up in bed and spending some time with Rich, normally watching total nonsense on television but nevertheless spending time with him. Going to bed early felt like missing out. So I came up with my five minute rule – I go to bed and if I am still awake after five minutes I would get up again and live the life. Let my body decide was the motto, and guess what, so far not once did I get back up.

Rich has to go to work in the morning and I try not to get him involved unless I really have to. My magic sleep number is six – if I get six hours of sleep per day, I am fine. I don't really need or expect a whole night's uninterrupted sleep, I don't mind being woken now and then, as long as I somehow get an accumulated amount of six hours I can conquer the world. But some nights you simply don't get much sleep, may it be down to teething, colds, tummy bugs or nightmares. Sometimes I find myself looking at the clock at 4am realising that I actually haven't really slept much yet and the night is nearly over. The morning after is tough but there is really no point stressing about it as stress won't change it for the better. I resort to taking it as easy as possible, stick to the bare necessities, get some daytime sleep, maybe shout for help and have an early night.

I try to catch up on sleep whenever possible, ideally when they both have a nap at the same time. Synchronised daytime sleep is really something to strive for, not only can I catch up on sleep or take a break, if I feel like it, I also get some jobs done or prepare dinner. Sometimes I take the girls for a walk, they fall asleep in the buggy and I then leave them in the buggy in my hallway and quickly have a nap. Sometimes I am lucky to find someone to look after them for an hour or take them for a walk.

After a while I started to put them to bed at a certain time, close the curtains, turn on their glow in the dark lullaby seahorse, maybe stick around a bit and then they would just sleep. The better their daytime sleep went, the easier was the night, which also made total sense.

But some days after a particularly rough couple of nights or when one or both were unwell, the girls simply didn't fancy a little synchronised sleep performance or one decided not to sleep at all or only in my arms whilst being carried around. This of course can be very lovely one to one time but when you are just desperate for a bit of sleep or a break it's not that appreciated. Those days I used to just accept being pretty exhausted by the end of the day. Understanding what sleep deprivation was doing to me, played an important role, I used to rest whenever I could; healthy food and plenty of fresh air helped to feel better. It also helped to talk to other mums, who were shattered too, or to post something on the internet and read the caring comments that follow.

> *"Sleep deprivation is regarded as torture under international law and is branded as such by the United Nations. Sleep deprivation [...] is an extraordinarily cruel form of torture which leads to a breakdown of the nervous system and to other serious physical and psychological damage".*
> *International Society for Human Rights (ISHR)*

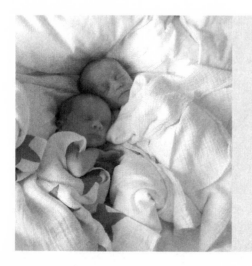

Who said torture?
Pure bliss!
Brad and Ellie
in dreamland.

Sleeping in separate beds

When I was 19 I went round to my then-boyfriend's house and realised his parents had their own bedrooms and I just thought "how weird is that?" Surely they no longer loved one another. He explained that this was the only way either of them would get any sleep and that they are still very much loved up. I didn't believe it. Surely they were secretly having affairs and sneaking other people back home into their own bedrooms. Well, I was 19.

I would have never believed I'd ever not share a bed with my husband for a prolonged period of time. That was until I was seven months pregnant with twins and I just couldn't sleep at night. I had to raise the head end of my bed so I would sleep in a near sitting position as I kept feeling dizzy when I was lying down plus it seemed to be the only position to keep the heartburn at bay. Luckily my bed does that sort of stuff. Towards the end of the pregnancy I really had to push myself up and out of bed, rolling over to the side before getting on my feet in order to take myself to the toilet every hour or so. I was really tempted to install a big rope to hang from our ceiling so I could pull myself up. Rich wasn't getting any sleep at all and moved into the spare bed.

When the girls were first born and we finally left hospital we moved back in with one another into our lovely marital bedroom, two Moses baskets on stands in front of the bed, expressed milk ready so Rich could bottle feed Jess whilst I breastfed Isla, quickly wind and change one baby each and then cuddle up together in bed with two stuffed sleeping beauties snoring their heads off whilst we whisper sweet nothings into one another's ears. Ha ha! We didn't whisper, it was more like shouting: "You didn't wind her properly." "Do you really have to switch the light on? Mine was fast asleep." "No, I don't know where the wet wipes are." - Total disaster. No one was sleeping or cuddling and nothing was done quickly and we were bickering in the middle of the night. Isla and I moved into the guest room. Rich carried on a few more nights' bottle feeding Jess but started to struggle getting up in the morning and having a long day at work. After a few nights I also noticed that my milk supply couldn't keep up with the demand, it was silly what we were trying to do, I just had to breastfeed both of them at night, I did it in hospital, surely I could do it at home, they were big enough to tandem feed which saved a lot of time anyway, so that's what I did. I moved both Moses baskets onto the guest bed, when one woke I'd wake the other, put them on my brilliant easy2nurse feeding pillow, wind them, change their nappies and place them back in their baskets.

The first months I managed to get around 90 minutes sleep, later on up to three hours and as long as I went to bed at around half past 9 / 10 o'clock I would normally end up with a total of around six hours sleep and that was fine. Once Jess and Isla had moved into their own bedroom we tried sharing a bed again but I'd still get up at night to feed them etc. and kept waking Rich or he'd wake me when leaving for work early, even though I could have done with another hour of sleep. Same for going to bed, I was ready to hit the pillows by 10pm when he just wanted to watch the news.

The bed wasn't the place where we'd kindle romance, we had plenty of that on the couch, the bed was really just the place where we'd desperately try and sleep. And it wasn't working. This time Rich moved downstairs into the guest room and that's where he still spends most nights now, two years later. It just works for us.

Every minute of sleep is precious; it's like gold dust to us. I can't enjoy my days if I don't get enough quality sleep at night. Same applies for Rich. I'd even go as far as to say that it adds a degree of excitement to our relationship. Some people tell us it's not good at all for our relationship so I read up on it and surprise, surprise, we are not the only ones, according to the US National Sleep Foundation, 23% of couples in 2005 slept in separate bedrooms! Research by sleep scientists at Britain's leading sleep lab has shown that sharing a bed causes 50% more sleep disturbances. Those 50% combined with the sleep disturbance caused by our children probably would have taken us up to 99.9% and sleep was just way too precious to mess around like that.

I also read that in ancient Rome the marital bed wasn't at all for sleeping but for sexual congress, now that's something they don't tell you in history lessons. I think as long as you maintain physical closeness and romance in other ways, it's ok to sleep apart in order to protect your relationship, health and sanity during times like these. For now it's the best way! (I must add that by the time I finished this book we were back in the same bed but always kept the spare bed ready just in case our bed was getting too crowded.)

ALCOHOL WON'T HELP YOU(R) SLEEP!

We all know alcohol induces sleep, it makes us sleepy, makes us pass out in pubs, on pavements or in the wrong bed. :) It's an adult thing we seem to enjoy after having spent a whole day with small children, it's what we had to hold back on whilst pregnant or breastfeeding and it relaxes us. But it also messes with our quality of sleep: big time. Recent studies confirm that alcohol induces sleep and we enter deep sleep faster and longer but it has a negative impact on the ever so precious REM (Rapid Eye Motion) sleep.

So here is how it works: Sleep is a natural state of reduced consciousness needed for the growth and rejuvenation of our body's immune, nervous, skeletal and muscular systems.

Our sleep goes through phases of non REM (NREM) and REM sleep. REM sleep occurs around every 90 minutes and dominates the latter half of sleep. It's during REM sleep that we have memorable dreams and are completely paralysed. A serious lack of REM sleep is linked to depression and the inability to deal with complex tasks. Naturally our

REM sleep is battered and beaten when we have little children, but you just have to cherish every little bit you're getting. When sleep deprivation kicks in the idea of a few glasses of wine or some beer might appear to be a good plan to help you relax or switch off. Its consumption will most likely induce sleep but at the same time it suppresses REM sleep as we can only enter REM sleep once our blood alcohol is down to zero. It also lightens NREM sleep.

Doesn't sound good for someone like me who really needs every minute of quality sleep they can get. I am not telling you to go teetotal- I just found that it really wasn't the wine I was after anyway, I was after that feeling of having an adult drink, something other than water. So we started making up non alcoholic cocktails or different types of tea. Having a variety of juices, lemonades and sparkling waters in the house is ideal. Ice cubes or mint leaves make any drink more special. A pint glass of half sparkling water, half apple juice looks just like a pint of beer but is way more refreshing. Just some ideas: Cheers!

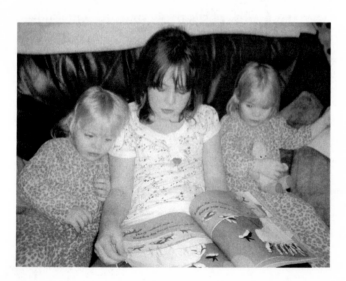

Big sister Lily reading a bedtime story to her twin sisters Heidi and Sophie.

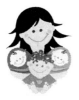

Older Siblings

Older siblings need to go to bed too, that's a fact. And they would also like a bed time story, milk, a cuddle, be tucked in, music on, lights off, tucked in once more, one more story, locate favourite teddy, kiss, one more story...

Jacob was sleeping perfectly happy in his racing car bed before his twin sisters arrived. He didn't really come into our bed any more, maybe once a month after a bad dream or when he wasn't feeling well. This all changed when the girls arrived. He pretty much spent the entire first three weeks after his sister's arrival in daddy's bed. When the girls and I finally came home, we tried to convince him to sleep in his own bed again but he said he felt lonely. He started waking up at night as he had a lot of "bad dreams" and the babies' cries woke him from time to time.

It appears to be quite common that a perfectly happy sleeping toddler suddenly starts waking up at night when siblings arrive.

I found myself expecting too much of Jacob, after all he was only three years old, but he just suddenly looked like such a big boy when those tiny babies arrived. He could walk, talk and sleep in his own bed and with his sisters being up so much at night, I was kind of expecting him to at least be "good" and stay in his own bed. We explained to him how much we loved him and how great it was that he was able to understand that he sleeps in his own bed and how silly it was of Jess and Isla not to like their lovely cots. We got him to check their cots in the dim light to see if there was anything scary and then we made some changes. I asked him to choose some lullabies to play to the girls at bedtime and asked him to explain to them that mummy and daddy are always just next door and there was really no need to cry at bedtime. He was the big boy helping his little sisters to sleep and he soon was happy again in his racing car bed. He sometimes climbs into bed next to daddy in the morning but I think it's mainly to grab hold of the iPad!

When the girls were eight months we moved Jacob into their bedroom, mainly as he was still complaining about being lonely and also in order to make bedtime easier. The plan was to read bedtime stories to all three children together and then put them all to bed at the same time. My friend Charlotte has four small children and that's how they do it every night but it didn't work for us. We managed for a few weeks, and it was really sweet, Jacob was singing lullabies to his sisters and all was good until the next tooth appeared and the girls started waking Jacob at night. So Jacob moved back into his own bedroom and we were back to two separate bed time missions. I soon realised that I couldn't spend hours putting the girls to bed whilst Jacob was waiting, parked in front of the television so mummy could sort out those noisy twins. I had to set a limit to the fuss upstairs. The girl's bed-time soon established at 7pm and Jacob's bedtime at 7:30pm. It works most days.

Glimpse into the future

What a difference some sleep makes! **My girls are eight months today** and I am finally getting somewhere. They both slept through the night last night and the night before and I slept like a rock and now I feel on top of the world. I hadn't written a single page during the last three weeks as some nights I only had 90 minutes sleep throughout the entire night (in three chunks of 30min that is) and I felt too drained to write a single line. But now I am back!

Jess and Isla are ten months now and night times are a challenge at the moment but you've just got to love the daytime: they are really starting to interact with one another.

They are so happy when they see each other in the morning and gently touch their twins' face. Then they go over to steal the other one's toy, dummy and food as that's so much more fun. I "found" them both in the hallway yesterday and they were looking at a picture together and somehow chatting away – so cute! Makes you forget all those sleepless nights.

At three years the girls are now in toddler beds. We first positioned them apart from one another on different walls but soon pushed them next to one another as this makes bedtime stories much easier and they seem to sleep much better this way. One of them will normally try and negotiate another story or announce that it's too early for bed but we just reassure that it really is bedtime, kiss and cuddle them and leave the room and they normally chat a little bit or sing and then they fall asleep.

They still occasionally wake at night, for example to go to the loo and sometimes I automatically take them back to my bed only for them to tell me that they want to go back to their own "princess bed". One of them ends up in our bed around once a week, which is fine.

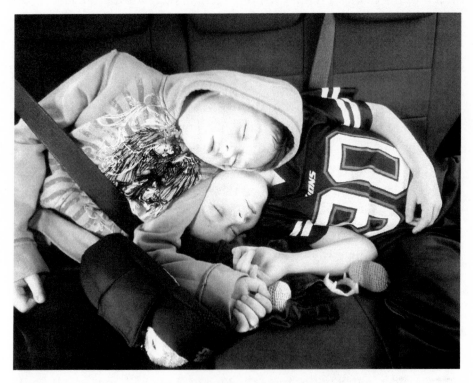

I just love this photograph of eight
years old twin brothers Hank and
Elvis, fast asleep on the backseat of
their car.

{CHAPTER 4}

COPING WITH CRYING

Dogs bark – babies cry.

Hearing someone's new born baby cry is kind of cute, hearing your own babies cry at 3am when you've done everything you can possibly think of and all you want is to just sleep: not so cute! Your 20 months old twins rolling around on the supermarket floor, crying their eyes out because you didn't allow them to drink the washing up liquid you just placed in your full shopping trolley: Not cute either. But let's start at the beginning.

Babies generally cry because they are hungry or thirsty, uncomfortable, in pain, ill, scared, bored, frustrated, in desperate need of a big cuddle or a random combination of the above. In order to find out what is actually wrong it helps to have some sort of system. I used the Cry-Sis checklist. Cry-Sis is a charity dedicated to coping with crying and they kindly granted permission to publish the list at the end of this chapter. The list is great but I think it's also important to acknowledge that just being a baby, growing physically and mentally at such a fast pace is reason enough to cry. Therefore I am going to tell you a bit about mental growth spurts and the development of the brain as I find this knowledge very reassuring and calming.

"Sometimes I just need a cuddle. I dont have a tummy ache, a growth spurt or a new tooth. I simply need someone to give me a cuddle and make me feel safe." Your baby

When the girls were little I kept reminding myself that they simply have no way of communicating other than crying. They simply can't talk or text, tweet or write on my Facebook wall, all they can do is cry and in the beginning they are not even good at crying, but I could count myself lucky as I had plenty of opportunity to study their cries and master the fine art of figuring out what they are trying to say, plus with time and a lot of practice they would be getting better and better at crying too. As easy as that! Yeah right, not simple at all and not the nicest subject to study, but it did pay off to just not panic when they cry but to listen and remember and to gradually work out what they want.

Whilst working my way through the list of reasons why my ba-bies were crying I used to try and stay calm, redirect my focus to some music, sing a song, take lots of deep breaths and repeat the following sentences over and over again, and I know it might seem odd reading them if you haven't had your twins yet, but trust me, one day these sentences will make sense:

- This is a bad moment but we have a million wonderful moments too. This moment will be over soon.

- The crying will stop.

- Don't take it personally. They are not crying to upset me.

- They are asking me to help them.

Sometimes it was just impossible to stop the crying and at times I got really stressed out for not being able to work out what they were crying about. But maybe they didn't even know it themselves. It happens to all of us now and again, that we simply don't know what we're whinging about. Just imagine you were out shopping with your best friend , she's in a foul mood because her partner forgot their anniversary plus she's convinced her bum looks big in pretty much everything she tries on. She complains all morning, and what do you do? You give her a hug and make her a cup of tea, and it will help even though that's not what your friend is crying about.

One evening my husband came home after work and I gave him an update about how much the babies had cried and how much our three year old had been whinging and he said: "I can see where they get it from" and I realised that actually I might be worse than all three of them together. So I came up with the whinge multiplier to see who whinges more, myself or my babies. As an adult I am obviously able to understand why I cry, I can communicate it and I can do something about it, plus I am old enough to understand that I just don't scream in public. My babies can't. Using my whinge multiplier of four, every one of my whinges translates into four minutes of them crying. I kept track of my beloved comments such as "Oh I am so tired" or "I wish they would stop crying" and guess what; I won the whinge world cup!

This all doesn't sound too bad does it? But it can get worse, if the crying hits you when you are tired and irritable and you might find yourself stuck in the house on your own, both babies crying, you're not dressed, they aren't either. You can't think, your brain is just not working... the crying gets to you, you're tired and can't work out

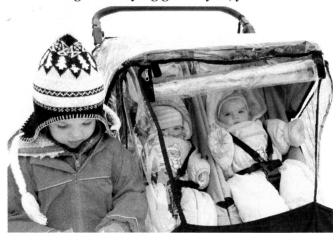

Out for a walk - come rain or shine!

what to do and all you want is to just get out!

And that's what you should do! Get everyone out of there and go for a walk. A walk always helps. I always had my buggy ready!
Some blankets or all in one suits were all I needed. The babies did calm down and so did I. Who cares what you wear, as long as you wear something. Flip flops in the rain are perfectly suitable footwear as feet will dry again: plus nobody looks at you anyway; they all just look at your babies. If my babies were overtired they would fall asleep. If they were bored before, they were now entertained.

If the crying didn't stop, at least I took the opportunity to clear my head and think of my next move, what could I try when I get home, is there anything I hadn't checked yet? Who could I phone and ask for help? It's such a simple little trick but it really helps to just take a deep breath when feeling all worked up and to only think of the next step. Tell yourself: "I will make it through the day, the week and the whole year and they will stop crying, they really will."

ADULT TIME-OUT

Please note: This might not be a subject you want to read about whilst you're pregnant but it nevertheless is a very important subject!

One day I had a conversation with a few fellow mums about that horrible feeling when you've run out of patience and feel like flogging your children on eBay, any offer accepted. Too much crying, not enough sleep, total exhaustion, whatever the circumstances exactly are: They have led to a point where you have simply had enough.

Normally this happens when the little one can't be settled and keeps crying despite all efforts to soothe him. We established that it often seems to be down to teething or baby being overtired and even though another day you would just stay calm and deal with it, some days you get stressed, upset and frustrated. When you have done everything you can think of and you find yourself getting angry with your child, then it might just be time for some adult time-out. Your baby needs to be in a safe place such as his cot and you need to pull the emergency cord and calm down. Your baby might even fall asleep whilst you take a deep breath. Phone someone if it helps; ask a friend to come over if possible, listen to music, eat chocolate do whatever helps to calm you down.

I wondered what help really stressed parents could find in my local area and found a weekly group for mums led by a health visitor, with a crèche facility. They kindly allowed me to come along to one of their meetings. There was an egg timer sat on the table and everyone got ten minute talk slot. Mistreating the children and the guilt connected were the number one issue. One of the ladies described in tears how awful she felt for having shouted at her baby when she just wouldn't go back to sleep at night. She said: "I shouted at her and she smiled back at me as she was so happy to see me. I felt like a monster." When it came to my ten minute talk slot, I really worried about what I could talk about. But the minutes just flew by and even though there wasn't much bugging me, I felt really liberated after sharing my thoughts about my sleepless nights.

Anger was mentioned a lot. Anger is an awful feeling. I came across Scott Noel's parenting website www.scottnoelle.com. Scott writes about transforming anger:

"Anger always arises from a perception of disempowerment. This must be a misperception because who you really are is truly powerful! Once you make peace with your anger, you can harness its energy and use it creatively."

Rather than being angry with your children, have a go at that anger building up in you. Tell that stupid anger to leave you alone and to stop messing around with you. Redirect its energy and go for a long walk.

BABY BRAINS

We know so much about our babies' bodies, but yet so little about their brains, despite the major influence of brain development on our babies' behaviour and the influence of parenting on the development of our child's brain.

Not only does the brain triple in size during the first three years of life, the crucial connections between the different parts of the brain are formed. Parents can actively influence the so called "Integration" between the logical left side of the brain and the emotional right side of the brain. We can help our children to thrive socially, emotionally and intellectually. Many tantrums for example develop when the emotional side takes over and the bridge between both sides of the brain hasn't been developed – but this is actually when the bridge is being built. It's during these situations when you naturally feel like using distractions to avoid the tantrum or ignoring your child during their rant, that you can actively help them build the bridge and integrate the different parts of their brains.

The book The Whole Brain Child by Dr. Daniel J. Siegel, M.D. and Dr. Tina Payne Bryson, Ph.D. explains all of this and also how you have to address the captivators' side of the brain first and then move over to the other side. For example if your child loses the plot as they wanted to open the last (!) yoghurt by themselves, without mummy's help, then there is absolutely no point in explaining that it really doesn't change the taste of yoghurt and that it was the last one, as the logical side of the brain is simply unaccounted for. So you approach the side in charge first, giving them a hug saying: "I know you really wanted to open the yoghurt because you are so good at it. It's such a shame." And then gently bring some logic into the game for example by checking if it had any impact on the taste of the yoghurt. I just love this knowledge! It also really helps to stay calm and accept meltdowns, take them for what they are, not a battle between parent and child but the building of a bridge.

It's a parenting opportunity but at the same time can be a really stressful situation, especially when in public, or when tired or in a rush to get somewhere.

MENTAL LEAPS

We have all heard about growth spurts, suddenly babies feed continuously and outgrow all their clothes at once. But they also go through mental growth spurts, called mental leaps. During these mental leaps they learn to understand the world around them. Suddenly their brains are able to comprehend something new, something they simply weren't capable of perceiving before. Examples are the understanding that our world is made up of certain patterns, relationships and sequences. Suddenly it is funny if a cat jumps up or a tower of blocks falls over, because your babies have learned that it's unusual and not the normal pattern.

The Dutch psychologists Hetty van de Rijt and Frans X. Plooij have spent over 35 years studying mental development in children and they have found that all babies live through the same developmental leaps at the same time and that babies are clingy, cranky and cry more when they are about to make a major mental leap forward.

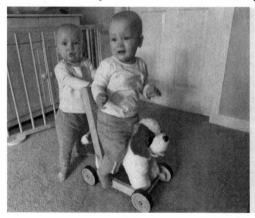

Hattie and Bea learning to take turns.

They published their findings in the book "The Wonder Weeks". I first read it when Jacob was born and it is amazing just how accurate it is. With Isla and Jess the leaps all started a few weeks later, which made sense given the girls were born at 35 weeks rather than their brother at 40 weeks gestation.

The book guides you through the ten phases of mental development and it comes with checklists so you can keep track of what happened when. It's quite a challenge keeping a diary with twins and The Wonder Weeks is a great alternative as you can utilise it to memorise all those firsts with the added bonus of understanding why your babies are being difficult. A very interesting book and a great help to cope with crying!

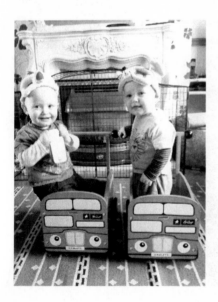

Another "milestone" met, we suddenly know how to drive a bus! Clever boys Hector and Felix.

HAVING UNWELL BABIES

"Prematurely born babies are much more likely to pick up infections" said the nurse next to me, whilst two doctors where rushing to find a vein on Jess's hands and feet for IV access. It was scary. I kept stroking her little face, she was barely awake and only whimpered with every failed attempt to get access. My husband was walking up and down the hall with Isla who was sick too but not this sick. Jess had bacterial and viral pneumonia plus another viral infection and she was very dehydrated.

Our then family doctor has an appointment system that requires you to plan your children's illnesses two weeks in advance in order to get an appointment or of course you could take them to the walk in clinic and "wait like everyone else". But seriously, how could I have done that with two vomiting babies with very high temperatures and a three year old in tow? Surely I would just exchange a few more bugs with other unwell people? Totally impossible and ridiculous. I had tried for two days to get seen, the second day I didn't even make it past the receptionist.

The following morning I phoned a different practice, got an appointment straight away and an hour later we found ourselves in the situation described above. And all the time I blamed myself for not doing something sooner, but apart from the obvious step of taking her to hospital what could I have done differently? How did she get so dehydrated? I hadn't slept in days; I was exhausted from all the crying, the constant cleaning and disinfecting of the floors, the huge pile of washing, the mess in my house, from trying to feed them and from all the worry.

Maybe I didn't realise quite how sick she had been. I did try and write down both their medications and temperature readings but not the fluid intake or count of wet nappies. I would not let this happen again, so I designed my own medical log, a sheet to help me keep track of medications taken, temperature readings and how much actually goes in and comes out of my children. I found it to be a really helpful tool when things got a bit hectic. It also aids you to provide exact information when seeking medical help. In order to avoid overmedicating I would take a note of any medicines given and then cross out the next however many hours until the next dose.

I know, it's basic maths, but when you're really stressed and shattered it turns out to be a helpful little trick. You just take a look at the time and the sheet and realise that you're not allowed to give the next lot quite yet. I find it very important to have the 24 hours of the day on the sheet, as this allows for easier management of when the next dose of medication is due or allowed.

You might want to create your own medical log, but just as a start, here's mine. I use separate sheets per child, I find it safer and it allows more space for additional notes. Visit my website lifewithtwins.co.uk for a printable version.

CHILD NAME:

	AM - afer midnight/ morning												PM - afternoon											
	01	02	03	04	05	06	07	08	09	10	11	12 noon	1	2	3	4	5	6	7	8	9	10	11	12mid night
Temperature																								
Painkiller																								
Painkiller																								
Antibiotics																								
Milk feed bottle ozs																								
Breastfeed minutes																								
Food intake (spoon full)																								
Vomiting																								
Diarrhea																								
Wet nappy																								
Soiled nappy																								

THE TERRIBLE TWOS WITH TWINS

Darling, shall we call the exorcist?

The terrible twos with two are quite something, having one baby rolling on the supermarket floor is awful enough and you need both arms to remove the drama-toddler from the public eye, two down is rather tricky and leads to one of those "I wish I was an octopus" moments. It also catches a lot more public attention than a run-of-the-mill singleton meltdown. But you can't stay at home forever and wait for them to turn into lovely tame three or four year olds, it's all practice and part of them finding their way, learning the boundaries and how (not) to behave.

My girls always used to lose it when just getting to the supermarket checkout, trolley full of food, empty fridge at home, regardless of how much I fed them during the shopping trip or how often I let them push the trolley or add items to the cart – they had to lose the plot just before the finishing line. So I quit big supermarket shops for a while and ordered online. Sometimes we have a babysitter for a couple of hours in the evening and my husband and I do a big food shop together, best night out ever!

I read a really good book called "Toddler taming" – it's brilliant, a very healthy and funny approach at dealing with our lovely little tamtrum-toddlers. The book helps to understand what children think and why it's so important for them to go through this developmental stage. The thing with any meltdown situation is, to remember that it might appear that you've failed at everything, you've lost control, the child is doing what it wants and running riot or maybe the child is possessed and one should call an exorcist! Or maybe opt for Super Nanny instead? But that's just silly and unnecessary, meltdowns are an important part of that little person becoming a decent big person one day, and that rolling, shouting and kicking mini is still your child, who loves you dearly and wouldn't do any of this if it wasn't for their confidence that their parent loves them no matter what.

NO, NO, NO, NO

You say it all the time (for a reason) and then they start talking and one of their first words is "no" – and as annoying as this can be, I figured that it's important they learn to say "no" as I do want them to say "no" later in life: "no" to bullies, "no" to drugs, "no" to strangers. It's my job to teach them when a lovely "yes" would be more appropriate.

TWIN FIGHT CLUB

I guess all siblings fight with one another for various reasons. Toddlers are over-protective of their toys, or whatever they perceive to be theirs. Pre-school children like to have a squabble over something silly like the car seat and primary school children are fighting for fairness and equality and find constant breaches in their parents' actions.

When different aged siblings fight, you can at least try and appeal to the older and wiser one to stop the fight. With twins it is different as there is no natural birth order boundary. Twins tend to have a very close relationship and are quite sensitive to each other's feelings and behaviour. As we all know, falling out with your nearest and dearest hurts the most. They share parents, siblings, toys, friends, bedrooms and are sometimes subject to comparison and competition. Squabbles and fights are unavoidable and a very important part of their development, but damn, are they challenging.

There was a time when Isla and Jess had just turned two years and they kept biting and scratching one another. There is not a single photograph where none of them had some sort of scratch or bite mark. It was so bad, we had to separate them and tell them not to hurt one another over and over again. Fighting over mummy was one of the most challenging situations. They eventually got the message and stopped injuring one another. At three years old they have the silliest arguments over totally pointless things, preferably in the car. But they are also the best of friends and really care for one another when one has a scratch or needs a hand with something.

I have collected some ideas how to deal with the twin fight club:
- Let them have some toys that they don't need to share.

- Assign car seats, sides in the buggy and label them with their name to avoid squabbles.

- Take turns, one week let one go first, for example on a ride on, next week the other.

- Criticise bad behaviour, not the child itself.

- Sometimes children just need a break from one another, a time out doesn't have to be a punishment but can be an opportunity to take a break and calm down.

- Keep your calm, intervene minimally and assist them in resolving their issues.

DISTRACTION – ONE OF THE GREATEST TOOLS OF PARENTING

Sometimes a tantrum just needs to be avoided at all costs, may it be a part of brain development or not. Once you've been a parent for a while you will start to see it coming, the tantrum, the meltdown, the drama and a simple attention diversion could just avoid the drama. Distraction does the trick. Shouting "Look there is a cat outside our window!", suddenly pulling a completely silly face, making a rude noise and then blaming your child or jumping up for no apparent reason looking all around for a mouse – It's all part of a great game called "Distraction."

Sometimes we surprise our children so much that they actually completely forget why their world was just about to come to an end. You just have to be crafty; it totally depends on the child and your imagination. I always have some small toys and something silly in my handbag, like a fake purse with old membership cards, a mirror or something that makes a noise.

Singing or silly dancing to music helps sometimes, especially if I get Jacob involved in the show.

Showing them photos or videos of themselves on my phone does the trick sometimes. The best one though seems to be the whole pulling a funny face trick. Once when Isla was picking a fight over a nappy change I pretended to smell one of her ever so stinky feet and

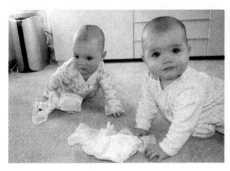

Who needs toys when you can play with clean nappies?

then pulled a face exclaiming "Yuck! Stinky feet." She loved it and kept holding out her feet for me to smell them over and over again whilst I changed her nappy.

Switching on the television is a proven form of distraction, for example when I just need to occupy them for a moment to get their milk or dinner ready. Also great are household items that aren't really a toy like wooden spoons, pots and pans, empty cereal boxes, empty yoghurt pots, anything that makes noises, let them rip up some catalogues (explaining that they can't do that with books of course) or put some pasta in little bowls and let them stir them.

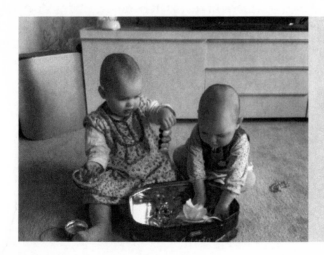

Best toy ever:
A biscuit tin
full of bangles.

BOREDOM AND FRUST

Babies and toddlers have an unbelievably s
least when it comes to activities we like the
be surprisingly persistent when they want
into a cupboard, but are easily bored when we want them to
five minutes in their playpen. I found that if I left them until they've
reached the end of their tether they'd get so upset that I would end
up spending a lot of time just calming them down. So I had lots
of "play stations" set up. I would for example place them on their
change mat for a while, then the playpen, then on a blanket on the
bedroom floor, then the baby gym on the lounge floor, bouncy chairs
in the kitchen and so on. Tidying toys away, so that they are out of
sight and only having a few out also really helped to keep them happy
and busy. Frustration also appeared to be playing a lead role in the
crying game. The girls couldn't wait to move about, they were getting
fed up, and it was like they were shouting: "I can't sit!   I can't walk!
I can't talk! But I really want to!"

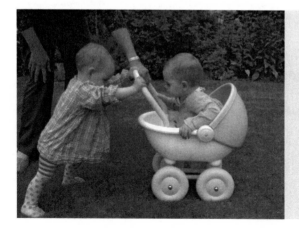

I can do it!

KERRI MILLER

SEPARATION ANXIETY

small children go through this stage, it's part of a healthy develop-ment and presents itself in your babies panicking and crying when you are out of sight even if just for a moment. It can start when babies are around eight months old and the stage lasts for some months and sometimes returns at pre-school age.

I couldn't even go to the loo without them as they got so upset when I left the room. And as every baby has to go through this stage, there are a lot of ideas how to make this stage easier on baby and parent. Read some ideas I have collected:

- When leaving the room, reassure them that you are still there even if they can't see you.

- When leaving them in childcare, tell them that you love them and that you will return to collect them. Keep your promises. If you promise to collect them before lunch, then do so.

- Have a good-bye ritual. Our ritual currently is "kiss, cuddle, pat " which my three year olds absolutely love as they are allowed to give us a very gentle pad when daddy leaves for work or when I drop them off at preschool. I can still hear them giggling when I am out the door.

- Keep on talking or singing when you leave the room so they can hear that you are still there.

- Time your departures after meals and naps and avoid leaving them when they are just due a sleep or a feed.

- Be patient with them, it won't last forever and no one will ever love your presence more than they do right now!

Older Siblings

When Jacob is in a good mood then he is my best helper when the babies cry, he is a little entertainer and soon distracts them if they are frustrated or bored. If Jacob isn't in the mood to entertain he would normally complain about the noise, hold his ears or join in. Those times aren't great and I would normally give Jacob something to distract him and then carry on calming his sisters.

My friend Rachael once told me about her daughter: "Freya has always been really loving to her brothers and would always cuddle them or try to entertain them if they were crying or entertain one if I was busy with the other. She was only two and a half when they were born but she has always been amazing with them. So loving and gentle."

Freya with her twin brothers Lukas and Malachi.

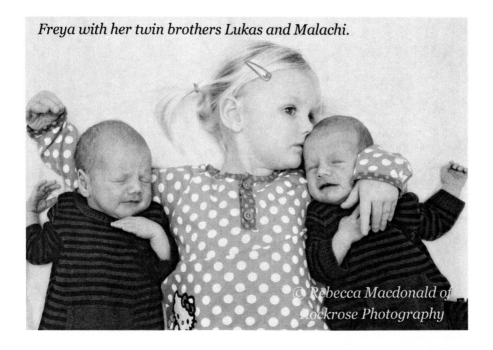

© Rebecca Macdonald of Rockrose Photography

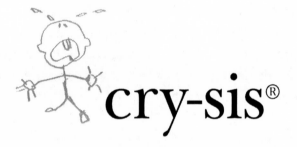

CRY-SIS® GUIDE TO COPING WITH A CRYING BABY

Introduction

The suggestions in this checklist are all ways in which parents have helped soothe their babies or coped with excessive crying. You may find that some of them work for you.

Is Baby Hungry?

- Offer breast or bottle feed

Is baby thirsty?

- Offer a drink from a sterilised spoon or bottle

Is baby in pain?

- Check for illness with G.P or Health Visitor

- Offer breast, bottle or dummy

- Offer cool boiled water or speak to pharmacist about infant colic remedies

- Try gently massaging baby's tummy in a clockwise direction

- Try changing baby's position

- Pick baby up, walk around with him/her – a baby sling can be helpful

- Try gently rocking baby up and down

Is baby tired but fighting sleep?

- Offer breast, bottle or dummy

- Try rocking baby horizontally in your arms or in a pram/pushchair

- Try a rocking or swinging cradle

- Try a quieter room

- Put baby down somewhere safe to cry for a short time – some babies settle themselves

- Try a softer light or a darker room

- Use a baby soother cassette or sing to your baby

- Quiet background noise can soothe babies – ticking clock, vacuum cleaner, washing machine etc.

- Check that baby is comfortable – clothes not too tight

- Check baby isn't too hot or cold – feel tummy to gauge temperature

- Motion can help babies sleep. Car rides or pram walks in the fresh air.

- A warm bath covering baby's tummy can be soothing

Is baby fighting at the breast?

- Check baby's position at the breast, most of your nipple should be inside the baby's mouth

- Check baby's nose is free of the breast (his/her head should be tilted back slightly)

- Check whether baby's nose is blocked and consult GP or Health Visitor accordingly

- Let baby suck on a dummy before quickly substituting breast

- Try changing feeding position, e.g. sitting up or lying down

- Is there too much milk? If so, express some off before feeds or feed on one breast changing sides at each feed for a few days

- Is there too little milk? Feed more frequently

- Consult Health Visitor, GP or a National Childbirth Trust (NCT) counsellor if you are still experiencing problems

Difficulty bottle feeding?

- Try a different bottle or teat

- Check the size of the teat hole and change to a different size if necessary

- Try offering bottles more frequently for a few days

- Leave for half an hour, and then try again

- Consult Health Visitor or GP

Is baby uncomfortable?

- Check baby's temperature by feeling tummy – adjust clothing accordingly

- Change baby's nappy

- Try different nappies

- Let baby kick, nappy-free

- Check for nappy rash – consult Health Visitor

- Check for clothing rashes

Sensitive baby?

- Handle and talk to baby gently and quietly

- Do not overwhelm baby with stimulation

- Try a quieter environment

- Try to keep to a routine and limit the number of visitors

Is baby generally cranky?

- Check for illness – consult Health Visitor or GP

- Talk to your baby

- Play with him/her: use toys or safe household objects

- Let baby kick, nappy-free

- Try using a baby sling to carry baby around

- Try a bouncing chair or baby bouncer (always follow manufacturers guidelines)

- Take baby out in pram or buggy

- Visit a friend

- Comfort by gentle rocking movement or soothing noises

- Offer baby a feed

- Massage baby and give warm bath

- Consult registered homeopath. Check with GP, Health Visitor

- Consult registered Cranial Osteopath with paediatric experience

- If you suspect Colic, speak to GP or Health Visitor about infant colic remedies

Still crying?

- Put baby down in a safe place, walk out of the room and shut the door, take a short break

- Give baby to a trusted friend or family member for a few hours if possible

- Use any time away from baby to look after yourself

- Eat well and unwind

- Go out with baby

- Phone your GP, Health Visitor, NHS Direct, The Cry-sis Helpline, friend or relative

Night-time Crying

Checklist and ideas for settling a baby under a year old

- Make sure baby is not hungry or thirsty

- Check that baby is comfortable and that his/her nappy is clean and dry

- Make sure clothing is not too tight

- Is baby too hot or too cold? Check baby's tummy temperature

- Rhythmic movement often settles babies. Gentle rocking in a pram or crib can have a hypnotic effect. Baby Slings are useful as they provide continual movement and the security of Mum/ Dad

- Some babies prefer the dark, others like a low night light

- Soother tapes and devices may help baby fall asleep. A bedtime routine is a worthwhile investment for the future. This is best introduced as soon as possible with perhaps a warm bath before bedtime and a quiet feed and cuddle before sleep

- From 3 months babies are becoming more aware of their environment, so other methods of settling them to sleep can be considered. Mobiles and soft play things above the cot prevent boredom and make baby's cot a more enjoyable place to be

- As baby gets older a particular toy or "cuddly" can be encouraged so that baby feels more secure when on his/her own. Soft toys in the cot can act as insulators – avoid overheating baby

- Many babies find their own fingers or thumbs to suck for comfort

www.cry-sis.org.uk

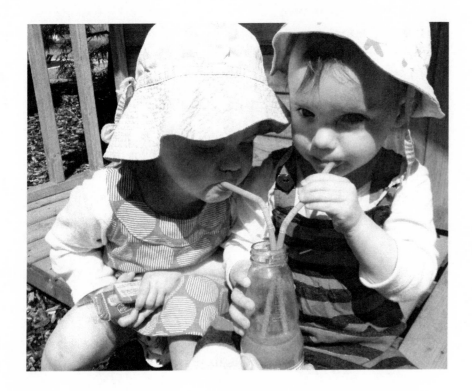

{CHAPTER 5}

CONFIDENCE WHEN FEEDING

All those night feeds. All the peeling, chopping and mashing. All the warming up of food followed by blowing to cool it down again. All those hours of feeding are rewarded by that great feeling that comes from watching your babies grow.

Mother Nature is a wonderful thing, you instinctively know that you need to feed your babies; breastfeeding on demand is a highly instinctive way of feeding a baby with your body creating the right milk for your babies' developmental stage.

But what if you bottle feed – how many ml per feed do your babies need? When do you start introducing solid foods? And which ones are suitable? And which ones are not? Motherly instinct simply doesn't tell you. Back in the day, new mums were more likely to have this knowledge as they may have grown up with plenty of family around them, maybe with babies in the same house. Nowadays we tend to have to work it out once our babies arrive. There isn't really much preparation during pregnancy other than the gathering of information about nursing.

Feeding can be stressful as it is a big responsibility, but talking to other parents and reading up on feeding helps.

Below are some great sources for information on breastfeeding, bottle feeding and the introduction of solids:

- **UNICEF** offers very helpful information on breastfeeding, bottle feeding and introducing solids. Visit their website and navigate to the parents section www.unicef.org.uk/ BabyFriendly/Parents/Resources/Resources-for-parents.

• **TAMBA** offers free leaflets and brochures covering all aspects of having multiples, including feeding them. www. tamba.org.uk

• Visit the **NHS UK** website on www.nhs.uk and navigate to Pregnancy and Baby, Your Newborn or to the Baby and Toddler section.

• **The Multiple Births Foundation** offers a great, free feeding guide which can be downloaded from the publication section on www. multiplebirths.org.uk

I breastfed for a year and started to introduce solids at six months of age. Breastfeeding my full term, singleton baby Jacob was a little challenging during growth spurts but all in all quite easy and effortless. Breastfeeding premature twins after a c-section with both of them in incubators and having to express every three hours – that was far from easy. I nearly gave up three days after birth, but fortunately it suddenly all fell into place and I carried on feeding both of them for a year.

But we all do things in our own way. Breastfeeding for a year was my way. Your way might be differently, because your life is most likely to be different from mine, so are your babies, your home and work circumstances. I have included feedback from other twin mums to demonstrate just how differently we all go about feeding our babies. There is no such thing as the "right way", only the right way for your family. One thing we all have in common though is that feeding baby twins is messy – really messy. But it is also incredibly cute! I will never ever forget those moments when they tried to feed one another, it was incredibly sweet.

*"Yes! You can breastfeed two babies. I did it, Sarah did it and
Lindy, Gitta and Emma are doing it right now."*

BREASTFEEDING

I have to admit that I am a bit crazy about breastfeeding. I am simply
amazed how clever the female body is, not only can we grow babies,
the service continues and our bodies create exactly the correct food
for our babies, no matter how small or large our breasts or nipples
are – they produce sufficient amounts of highly nutritious, antibody-
rich, easy to digest, just the right temperature milk straight from the
tap. Awesome!

I was always confident that it would be possible to breastfeed
two babies. It's logical really – the more milk your babies demand,
the more milk your body will supply! What I didn't know was just
how hard it was to establish breastfeeding premature twins and to
express for two babies. And I didn't expect how challenging growth
spurts with two babies could be. Please read my birth and hospital
diary starting from page 207 which includes all the details about how
we established breastfeeding with two babies in intensive care. By
the time I left hospital, Jess and Isla were both feeding well and I
loved breastfeeding! Especially as there was nothing to prepare, buy
and sterilise.

If you can breastfeed, then go for it! If you are not keen but
feel like you ought to, then at least give it a go! The health benefits
for yourself and the babies are undeniable, the precious antibodies
in your milk will give your children's immune system a head start
which premature babies really need and nothing else in this world
can replace. Plus it's so much easier to digest in their tiny tummies.
No powder can do what your milk can do.

I believe breastfeeding will make your life easier! You will never have the problem of overheating the boob or finding the nipple is still in the steriliser. You will never forget to bring your bottles or the bottle warmer; it's always there, on tap.

And not to forget the lush let-down feeling breastfeeding gives you, it's the reflex that draws the milk out of the storage into the nipple and releases the hind milk, in the early stages this will coincide with the cramping of the uterus (so called after pains) which is uncomfortable but a really important part of your body getting back to normal. Later on, the let down turns into a relaxing feeling. Many women describe that breastfeeding gives them a happy feeling which is scientifically linked to the release of the hormone Oxytocin aka "Love Hormone", a hormone described to evoke feelings of contentment, the ability to reduce anxiety, and creating feelings of calmness and security. Just what you need when you have baby twins.

The World Health Organisation (WHO): "Breastfeeding is one of the most effective ways to ensure child health and survival. Breast milk is the ideal food for newborns and infants. It gives infants all the nutrients they need for healthy development. It is safe and contains antibodies that help protect in-fants from common childhood illnesses. Breast milk is readily available and affordable, which helps to ensure that infants get adequate substance."

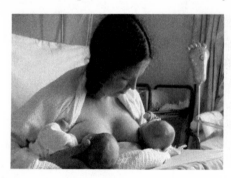

Gitta feeding her newborn baby girls on the double feeding pillow in hospital, gently holding their heads in place.

In the beginning I breastfed one baby at a time, which allowed me to concentrate on teaching her how to latch on properly and I could practise holding her in place. It's a steep learning curve, in no time we were well on the way and I moved on to tandem feeding. I tried with an ordinary breastfeeding pillow and a selection of random pillows at first but it was such a nuisance and one day Rich had had enough of the fuss and ordered a proper double feeding pillow and I never looked back. The pillow was amazing: U-shaped, foam filled and sturdy, slightly angled towards me so the babies would just roll into position and not fall off. It had a strap to secure it in place and also a wedge as back support. I would just "plug them in" and then I had both hands free to read a book, cuddle Jacob or use the remote control.

At night I took my pillow to bed with me and when they woke up I would feed them in my bed. I was feeding my babies in the so called rugby hold, something you can also do when feeding them individually.

At three months I was feeding them separately for a short while as they seemed to prefer the individual attention. Feeding them one at a time is very time consuming plus there is the chance you might leak from the side you are not using which is a waste of precious milk. I bought little plastic shells that I would slip into my bra to

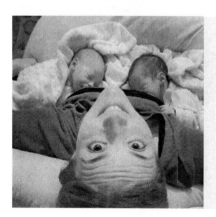

Twin mum Carmen tandem feeding her twins Max and Sofia. A brilliant photo taken by twin daddy Stephan.

collect any milk I was losing which was great when out and about as I would do pretty much anything to avoid those wagon wheel milk stains when in public. Very important was to remove the full shell when finished rather than tip it all over yourself when getting up.

And at four months we were back to tandem feeding as they started talking to one another and smiled at one another, one stroking the other whilst they were feeding. It was absolutely magical.

A book I found really helpful was *Mothering Multiples: Breastfeeding and Caring for Twins or More*, by La Leche League, Karen Kerkhoff Gromada. This book looks specifically into breastfeeding two babies, how to express for two and how to deal with all the stumbling blocks, for example blocked milk ducts.

I will always cherish the memory of them holding hands when I nursed them on my feeding pillow, such a very special time.

I really have my
hands full during "double winding".

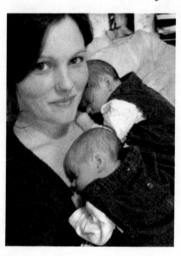
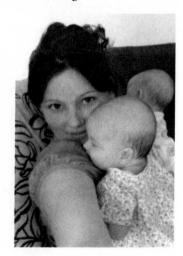

THE ART OF BREASTFEEDING TWINS WHEN OUT AND ABOUT

The obvious solution is to tandem feed at home with no one looking at what's on display and independently feeding them when out and about, only problem was that my two were usually hungry at the same time and one had to wait for the other to finish the feed. I felt

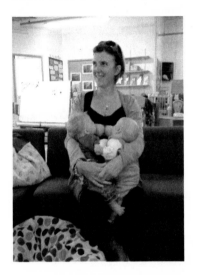

comfortable tandem feeding at twins club but not really in the park or at a soft play area. So I made one baby wait.

I wish I had thought of the ingenious solution demonstrated in the photo. All credits for this one go to my friend Emma, who found such a brilliant, easy solution to tandem feeding her twin boys in public without having too much on show - and she even let me photograph and publish it. Love it!

THE "I DON'T HAVE ENOUGH MILK" ILLUSION

If you ever feel like you don't have enough milk then that's because you don't have enough milk **at that very moment** but your body is already speeding up production and you will soon have more. Growth spurts can be difficult times as your body needs to speed up production and you might have thoughts such as "I don't have enough milk for my babies, they want to feed all the time, I have to stop feeding them".

Well, let's imagine you owned a restaurant; would you close your restaurant down just because your guests keep ordering more and more of your delicious meals? No way, you would just cook more! And that's exactly what your body will be doing, it will simply produce more milk, but you need to tell your body to "get back in the kitchen" and make more milk, your babies will do this for you by feeding and feeding and feeding.

I know it's very hard not to get stressed during growth spurts, but try to believe in your body, this incredible body that managed to build your babies in the first place! Your body will catch up and in a short while you will have enough milk to stuff your babies!

My friend Sarah once told me that she used to really struggle as she had too much milk for her singleton baby and used to flood the little girl. So her midwife told her to drink less and this apparently worked. All I could think of when listening to her story was that I wished I had the same problem. I would love to flood their little mouths, and so I started drinking much more. And I mean MUCH more! A pint of water during a feed and at least another one before the next feed was due. And it really did the trick. So simple and yet so effective!

Whenever I felt like I was "running out" or "didn't have enough milk" I would make a deal with myself to try for another two days before giving up. Two days later supply and demand were in line again and life got easier and I was glad I had tried a couple more days.

But when your confidence is shattered during a growth spurt or after a period of little sleep you might open up your heart to someone with little confidence in breastfeeding. They might tell you that your milk is not sufficient enough for your babies. Some mums say life got much easier once they stopped breastfeeding but maybe life would have been even easier if someone had helped them to carry on and they were still confidently breastfeeding their babies a little longer.

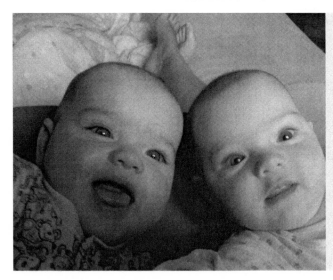

Come on mummy, we're ready for a feed!

When in doubt speak to someone who has knowledge about and confidence in breastfeeding, try and find a breastfeeding supporter or a lactation consultant or whatever they are called in your area. Speak to a health professional, ask other breastfeeding mums or contact La Leche group.

Maybe your babies are not latching on properly. Visit the Baby Friendly Initiative website to download their excellent feeding leaflet "Off to the best start", it shows great pictures of how to position your baby and a really well written explanation on how to latch your babies on.

www.unicef.org.uk/BabyFriendly/Parents/Resources/Resources-for-parents/Off-to-the-best-start

The main concern when a baby doesn't appear to be getting enough milk is poor weight gain. To check if your babies are actually gaining an appropriate amount of weight, it's always a good idea to see a health professional. For information purposes you can take a look at the World Health Organisation growth chart.

BREASTFEEDING WITH OLDER SIBLINGS AROUND

Some twin mums stop breastfeeding as they feel too trapped on the couch to look after older siblings. Jacob was already three when his sisters arrived and I always managed to keep him occupied when I fed them but I can see how this could be more difficult with a one year old who might be crawling off. Some ideas to keep them busy are to read a book with them whilst you feed the babies (totally do-able if you have a decent breastfeeding pillow), they could have a snack or feed their own teddies, do some drawing, watch television or have a special toy in their playpen or the travel cot. It just needs to be planned.

One twin mum I met through TAMBA bought a couple of toy babies for her first born daughter Gracie who was two years old when her twin sisters arrived. Whenever mummy fed the babies, so would Gracie, such a cute idea.

COMBINED BREAST / BOTTLE FEEDING

When I left hospital, my three weeks old twins were both happily breastfeeding and taking expressed milk from a bottle. I had expressed around ten litres of spare breast milk whilst Isla and Jess were tube fed. I tried to donate it to the special care baby unit but all the checks would have been much too costly for them. So they sent me home with a bag full of bottles which I used up by letting Rich feed the girls now and then or in order to go for a meal out with my husband. We'd leave the girls and a couple of bottles with granny and grandpa and whizz off for a couple of hours. Once the expressed milk was used up, we stopped the bottle feeds thinking they'd still be happy to take milk from a bottle a couple months later when we were invited to a childfree wedding party in a beautiful Devonshire castle. Well, they no longer wanted the bottle regardless of content, teat, temperature or who was feeding them. I think it would have been a good thing to carry on with a bottle once a week or so. But I didn't have to return to work and didn't need them to take milk from a bottle. I wasn't really expecting they'd go on a bottle strike just before the wedding. We did go to the wedding. I just had to drive home to feed Isla and Jess a couple of times and brought them along for the evening celebrations.

Many twin parents combine breast and bottle. There are lots of different ideas and strategies, for example giving a formula top up in the evening, expressing milk in the morning and using it to top up in the evening or replacing some feeds with formula. All these largely depend on the individual circumstances and the best way is to talk to a breastfeeding supporter or health professional as they have an effect on your milk supply and need to be carefully considered. We tried top up feeds before bedtime on a few occasions and the girls did sleep much longer than they would have done without.

UNICEF and the Multiple Births Foundation both offer plenty of information material.

IF BREASTFEEDING DOESN'T WORK FOR YOU

Some pregnancy and birth experiences make it hard or impossible to breastfeed, some conditions make it impossible to carry on breastfeeding and many mothers feel sad and disappointed. One thing to remember is that every drop of breast milk they've had has benefited their immune system and that there are several other ways to bond with your babies. The whole topic is only really relevant whilst you're going through it. It's a bit like all that talk about pregnancy and birth. In a few years time you will barely talk about how the birth went. You will be talking about pre-school, individuality and potty training.

If you are going to be bottle feeding, then just do it, move on, get organised, enjoy cuddles with your babies whilst giving them a bottle and also enjoy that you can share the responsibility to feed your babies.

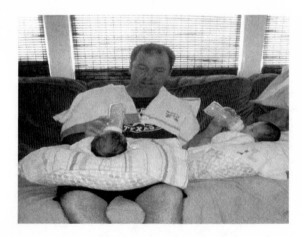

Very well prepared daddy Ben busy feeding his twins William and Isaac.

BOTTLE FEEDING

The majority of twin mums will bottle feed their babies at some point using either formula or expressed breast milk. This may be because breastfeeding didn't work out, returning to work or simply to have a meal out whilst someone else takes on a feed.

My bottle feeding experience is limited yet I have learned that you need to get organised when bottle feeding. Bottles need to be clean and sterilised in time for the next feed, water needs to be boiled and cooled and feeds prepared. You will need a sufficient amount of bottles and teats, a steriliser, age appropriate formula or expressed milk. If you express you might need a pump and freezer bags.

There are double feeding pillows available, an alternative are two kidney shaped pillows, car seats, bean bags, bouncers to sit your babies in whilst you feed, or have them on your lap of course.

You can buy special dispensers and pre-fill the sections with the right amount of powder in advance, which saves time and having to drag the whole pot of formula around. Including a time slot for sterilising and cleaning in your daily routine is often recommended. And as there is nothing more stressful than running out of food it's often suggested to keep a good supply of formula at home.

One approach is to prepare bottles with boiled, cooled water, scoop formula into dispensers and then mix the two when re-quired and then heat the bottle in a cup of warm water or using a bottle warmer. A few twin mums from my local twins club have managed to convince their twins to take their bottles at room temperature. Another alternative is to purchase liquid ready milk.

A collection of bottle feeding ideas:

"Get help with one baby whenever you can!...find a comfortable position when on your own where you can

feed both at the same time...and get them holding their own bottle as soon as possible, makes life a whole lot easier but always be close by for that all important eye contact and special bonding time. Also get daddy involved lots when bottle feeding, I know Daniel enjoyed the bonding experience a lot when I moved on from breastfeeding as before it was very much a mother and baby thing and now it was his time to have some special time with his babies."

Gemma, mum to Sophie and Heidi, Barrett

"I bottle fed from day one. At night my husband and I would feed one each, and during the day when I was on my own. I'd feed one then the other. After a while I realised how time consuming this was so fed both together in their rocker chairs. Two pairs of hands are always better than one but if you haven't got that luxury you'll find a way to improvise that works for you both. I found that if I asked someone to feed one of the babies they felt privileged to be asked. Don't be afraid to experiment with different formulas or bottles/teats, what agrees with one baby doesn't always with the other. I had one very hungry and colicky baby who would do some amazing projectile vomiting and muslin cloths were my saviour whilst bottle feeding."

Gillian, mum to Joshua and Oliver

"We bottle fed from as soon as they were home. If we were both home, me and their dad would feed one each but I had to find

ways to feed them both when on my own. I used to feed them one at a time when they first came home, mainly because they were so small I couldn't find a comfortable way of feeding them at the same time. It was more time consuming but luckily Ethan was very patient and would happily wait to be fed second. Once they got a little bigger I would put the bouncy chair one end of the sofa, feed one in there whilst feeding the other resting against my opposite arm. People used to ask how on earth I did it, but it was in fact very easy this way. As Gemma said above, it became even easier once they could hold their own bottles."
Zoe, mum to Ellis, Ethan and Sophia

"I bottle fed them from about two weeks old. When my husband was at home we fed them at the same time, which backfired a bit because when I was on my own they would cry at the same time and I could only feed one at a time until they were a few months old and Oliver could hold his own bottle (about eight weeks). It got easier especially once they didn't need the middle of the night bottle." Ingrid, mum to Oliver and Jack

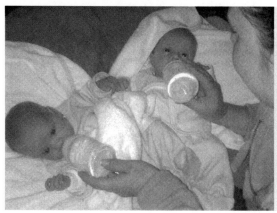

Twin Mum Nicolene bottle feeding her five weeks old twins Willem and Rulene.

KEEPING TRACK OF MILK FEEDS

Some days I couldn't even remember my children's names, let alone when they last fed. Maybe it's a habit I developed during our stay on the neonatal care ward, when we had to feed at a certain time and keep track of how long each baby had nursed for or how much expressed milk or formula they have had. I used an app on my phone to keep track of the feeds, it came with a stop watch functionality and would manage both babies, I would just switch to the correct baby, latch on, press "start" and "finish" and then set an alarm for in three hours time (not that I ever needed that alarm). It was pretty useful. It works for breast and bottle feeding as you could also enter quantities fed. It would also keep track of nappies, sleep etc. But a piece of paper also does the job! Keeping a log is a really useful idea, especially if you are alternating breasts and want to keep track of who fed where last!

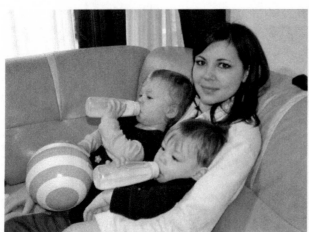

Olesea and her twins Karina and Kevin enjoying a little milk-break.

WEANING

I didn't even know what the word "weaning" meant until I got thrown into it when my first born started to want something other than milk. The definition of weaning is:

"To accustom the young of a mammal to take nourishment other than by suckling."

I would define it as making the biggest mess possible with food whilst using a small proportion of it for eating.

But what was allowed and how much? I didn't really know. Luckily there is a lot of info available, I suggest visiting the sources introduced at the beginning of this chapter.

I found Annabel Karmel's books very helpful. They come with a planner and various recipes for home made baby foods. This, of course, kick starts the desire to be the amazing mum who provides an array of beautifully home cooked meals but that's not always possible so I quickly found ready baby meals starting to fill up my shopping trolley and leaving a hole in my purse.

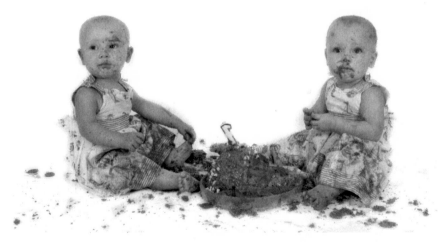

Hattie and Bea demonstrating the idea behind weaning.
© Celia Moore of Cherish Me Photography

Cooking my own meals worked out to be a lot cheaper, especially as babies waste a lot of food by using it as facial moisturiser and finger paint, but it took up a lot of time. So when I managed to cook my lovely home made foods using fresh and sometimes local fruit and vegetables I tried to make a big batch, freeze it in ice cube trays and once frozen, I would transfer the food cubes from the trays into bags so I could carry on using the trays. That way I would only ever waste small quantities, which was less heart breaking. Some of my friends went for Baby Led Weaning. It simply means letting your babies feed themselves with finger foods, rather than mashing, pureeing and spoon feeding them. Use an internet search for more info.

One day my friend Charlotte turned up with various freezer bags full of home made baby food. I was just about to run out when she knocked on my door. Those bags with mashed all sorts were one of the best presents ever!

Running out of baby food is not a good plan. I soon realised that I needed a large amount of food. I simply couldn't make all my own baby food and started stocking up on prepared baby foods. I once met a singleton mum at a breastfeeding group, who told me that she'd never ever feed her son any prepared baby foods but cook everything from scratch. She went on to tell about how she struggled with feeling very low for a while and felt incapable of cooking anything for her

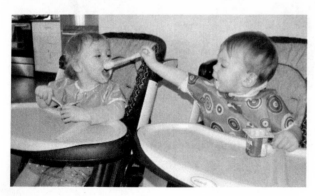

Kevin feeding his twin sister Karina.

son and therefore fed him on biscuits and milk for a week. I felt for her and her son, but didn't really agree with the concept that a week on biscuits would be a better idea than a week on baby food jars. As soon as I left the group I went to the supermarket to stock up on baby foods for Jess and Isla – and biscuits for myself.

Feeding six months olds is a huge mess! Their hand eye coordination isn't great yet but their desire to feed themselves is massive. They love touching and squashing their food, sucking on vegetables and smearing yoghurt all over their faces.

Here are some ideas I collected:

• Use one spoon and bowl for both (unless one is ill). It takes forever to feed them from two bowls using two spoons.

• Get high chairs with tables with a high rim or, if they are sat at a table, get dishes with a high rim, this helps to keep food on the plate/tray and helps the babies to grab hold of it.

• Get pelican bibs, they catch the food and your twins can finish off what's inside the bib.

• Place a mat under the table/ high chairs for easier cleaning.

• Have heaps of clothes / wet wipes to hand.

• If the room is warm enough, feed them topless.

• When they start climbing in and out of their highchairs: use harnesses or reins to secure them.

• Once they can sit, you could use a small table and chairs.

• Try offering their food unheated. It makes life much easier when out and about if food doesn't have to be a certain temperature for them to be happy to eat.

• Make a meal plan and then buy or order food accordingly.

- Some children love rice for breakfast, which is quick and filling and easy to combine with other foods such as grated cheese.

But some days they just don't sit down properly to eat. One day the girls were sat in their high chairs at our big family table and they just messed around with their food. They chucked most of it on the floor, ate absolutely nothing and then tried to climb out of the chairs. So I decided to try again in an hour or so, took them out of the high chairs and took some bits back to the kitchen. When I returned they were both sat under the table eating everything they had just chucked there. It had all landed on the clean mat I had placed under the table and high chairs and was fine to eat so I just let them go ahead. Some parenting experts might just throw their hands up in the air now and shake their heads in disapproval but it was so cute and most importantly, they were eating! No one was crying, they were actually cleaning up the mess they had made and, funnily enough, next time they sat nicely at the table, we didn't have to eat under the table for years to come and all was good. When they wouldn't eat properly, I tried making dinners a bit more interesting. I offered dips such as hummus and decorated their plates a little bit. Their favourite was "Dinner Mouse", which you can basically make up out of anything,

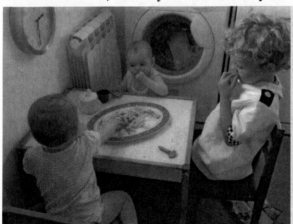

Snack time in my busy little kitchen.

a blob of mashed potatoes, baked beans ears, cucumber strip whiskers, carrot eyes and it could be hiding in some broccoli. Also very popular with my three are lunch boxes, they love to eat out of a lunch box.

Some days no lunch boxes or dinner mice could convince my children to eat, and they simply eat near to nothing, or at least I am under the impression they haven't had "anything to eat all day". One piece of advice I was given in this situation is not to look at how much they eat over the course of the day but over the course of a week. But it's such a waste to chuck all this food away; surely there was something I could do differently. They just didn't seem hungry enough. I asked my friend Sam, she has three boys and two of them have MCADD , a condition where the body is unable to break down certain fats, her boys have to eat their food or else they get very poorly. Sam would not give her children any snacks or milk an hour before the next meal was due as they wouldn't eat their meals. She would encourage them to stay at the table until they had eaten enough. She was incredibly strict and organised - she had to be. Well, I hadn't quite realised just how much my own children were

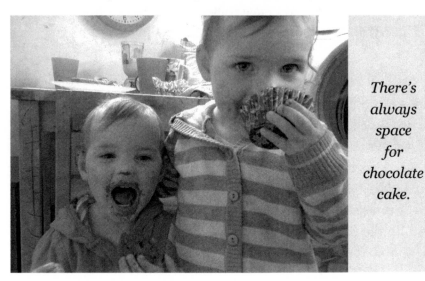

There's always space for chocolate cake.

snacking. I also found it helped, to give milk or any other drink after the meal. Having a meal plan is also a great tool, more about this in the next chapter.

Even with a fridge full of food, getting two or more meals ready can be quite a job if your children are very demanding at dinner time. Deciding what food to prepare or even how to prepare it was tricky when I had two little screamers attached to my legs. So one day I scribbled a list of easy to prepare, healthy fast foods and stuck it on my fridge. This was great. I would just pick something from the list, decision made. No more brain power required.

Some of these foods were:

- Muffin Pizza, slice a plain muffin and then add some tomato puree or actual tomatoes, grate some cheese on top, in the oven for a maximum of a couple of minutes. Done. If frozen I would just toast them quickly before adding the toppings.

- Vegetable sticks, bread and a pot of hummus. Messy but very quickly served.

- Pancakes, I always have some in the freezer (same for sliced bread) and the kids can add their own filling.

Now all I had to do was to free my arms and legs in order to get food ready. Sometimes a box of toys on the kitchen floor did the trick and distracted the girls enough to let me get on with dinner.

Whenever the toys didn't do the trick and there was some little monkey clinging on to my leg not letting me get dinner ready, I would place her in the travel cot, frequently called 'the trouble cot'. Her twin sister would normally just stay with her and either pass toys into the cot or cry alongside the travel cot and as harsh as this may sound, these situations only ever lasted for a few moments and were down to both of them being hungry.

My friend Cassie had a child gate at the kitchen door so her twins could see her but not stop her from preparing their food.

It's not just that you physically can't get anything out of cup-boards or cut food when you only have one hand or even no hands available. It's simply not safe if you are handling knives, pots and pans.

When I was out and about I sometimes used food pouches. I never warmed them up, the girls didn't mind if baby food was warm or cold. I collected all the tops as they looked way too cool to be thrown away. We used them to craft a massive rocket which is now hanging up in Jacob's bedroom. I never left the house without snacks. Bread sticks, some cut up fruit and a pot of boiled pasta were

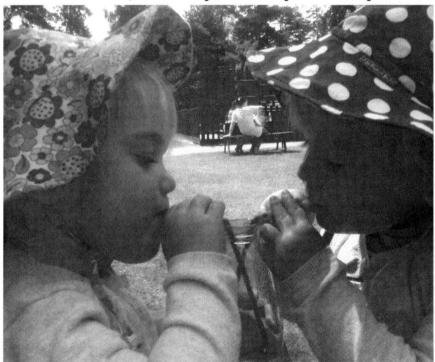

*Sharing is second nature for
twin sisters Jess and Lily.*

Glimpse into the future

my usuals.

My girls are **nearly six months old** whilst I am writing these words, I have started weaning them, I still breastfeed and have also started to give them solid foods such as carrot and banana. Jess is taking very well to real food, she gets really excited when she sees any, Isla is less interested, she eats some but she eats like she breastfeeds, very slowly and she kind of eats backwards, food appears to disappear and reappear rather a lot - messy but very cute.

Jess and Isla are nine months old

Oh what has happened to my life? It's 8am, I am sat in the kitchen with my 500 children, pardon, my three children. Isla is on solids-strike and hanging on my left boob, I am spoon feeding a "starving" Jess with my right hand and at the same time telling my three year old not to dance on the chair but to eat his breakfast instead, only to see him jump off the chair and running for the bathroom shouting "I need a poo!" And to top it all off, it's half term and I have a whole week just like this ahead of me.

Isla and Jess are three years old and I no longer stress about dinner. They eat what we eat and it's not such a big deal if dinner is served up half an hour later than usual. I still really try and stick to regular meal times though and avoid any snacks before the main meals as they still get rather grumpy when over hungry.

All three of my children eat school dinners without any complaints now, which is great as I don't need to make up two or sometimes three lunchboxes. They are suddenly interested in trying new foods and therefore it's become good fun to take them out for a meal now and again. Life is good!

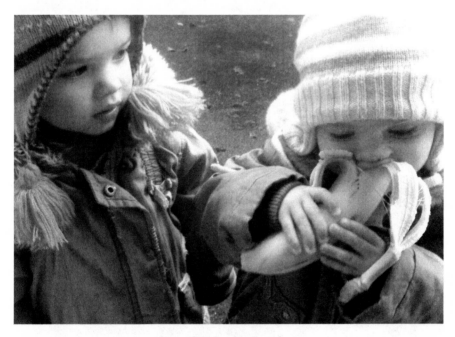

My cheeky little Isla
enjoying a banana.

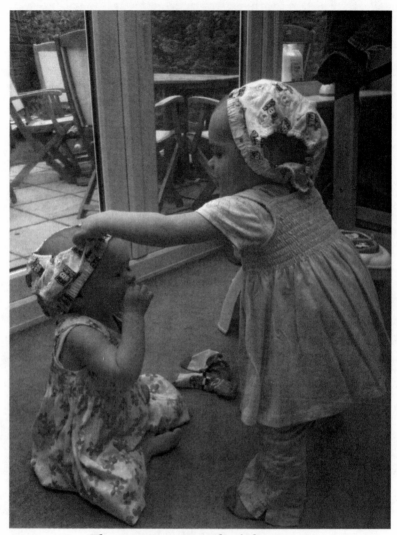

*There you go, now that's how you
wear boy's pants.*

{CHAPTER 6}

MANAGING YOUR NEW FAMILY LIFE

"Do more with less."
Ōhno Taiichi, 1912 – 1990

"We will be so outnumbered!" was my second thought whilst staring at the two little heart beats on the screen. I had to become more organised, for sure. Two adults, one toddler, two babies, two cats, a household, jobs, so many mouths to feed – that's a proper little family business and it needs some degree of management.

Whilst studying for my degree in Business Management, we talked a lot about Lean Management. You might have come across it before as it's a way of thinking which has been applied not only to businesses but also health organisations, schools, and the government in order to minimise waste and to make the most of what you've got. (Keep on reading, this is not turning into some boring business lecture, I promise.)

Let me introduce you to Taiichi Ohno , a Japanese businessman considered to be the father of the Toyota Production System, the first Lean Management System. Ohno found "Seven Wastes" which can be found in any process, for example the process of caring for baby twins. Anything you do: Think lean in order to eliminate waste and to do more with less! Use the least amount of time, money, effort[1]   and energy, equipment, facilities and materials – whilst giving your family (your customers) exactly what they need. Let's take a closer look at some them:

MAKE THE MOST OF YOUR TIME

Time was (and still is) my most critical resource, I constantly ran out of time. Whenever I visited either of my friends Sarah and Sam, whom I secretly call the "immaculate housewives", it was then when I realised just HOW messy my house was and I blamed not having enough time. I asked them how they found the time to keep their houses so pristine, both answered that they constantly clean and tidy up and that it never really gets untidy in the first place. But they both ENJOY it, I don't.

So this wasn't going to work for me. Yes, tidy up as you go sounds logical and I was trying to do that anyway, but a house as lovely and tidy as theirs was just not achievable. I was so busy with breastfeeding and later on with preparing dinners, it all took up so much time. Nappy changing, dressing, helping Jacob with his toys and crafts, come evening I had been busy all day and yet I felt like I had achieved absolutely nothing. That's silly and I know that but still, I always wished I had done more in the household. Sometimes Rich came home at the end of his working day and was a bit disappointed that we had actually managed to create even more chaos throughout the day. On one occasion, when the girls were six months old, he said "Well just tidy up as you go, don't create the mess in the first place." Well, let's not talk about the argument that followed.

I did not enjoy the chaos either but "tidy up as you go" is easier said than done and some days are more difficult than others, mainly as you need hands to tidy up and I never seemed to have any free

---

1 This is not to be understood as making less effort with your children but as in finding a more effortless way.

hands available. It was silly. One afternoon we all went to the beach somewhere in Cornwall and an older couple approached us. They said seeing our family reminded them of themselves a mere 40 years ago, when their own twin girls and toddler boy were the same age. The lady told us how she used to spend all day long playing with them, teaching them and fully concentrating on them. Then they both went on to explain how they had very fond memories of both of them putting the kids to bed together at the end of his working day and then spending the following hour tidying up, cooking dinner and catching up on one another's life and the world in general. I could have kissed them both! So when the babies were little this is what we did. There were some days when I managed to get more jobs done, this was either because they slept at the same time or later on when they started to entertain themselves a bit more. But even then I soon came to realise that I simply didn't have enough time to do everything that COULD be done but the good news was that with a little bit of management I was able to have enough time to achieve everything that NEEDED to be done. I felt it reduced my stress levels and made me feel more in control. Plus it also made life easier on those days when I felt like doing nothing or when the babies were unwell.

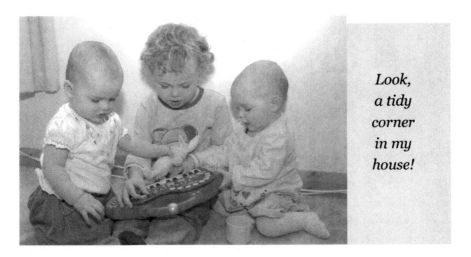

Look, a tidy corner in my house!

The fact is you can't do everything, in the long run you will have to give up a few activities that you used to do before you had 500 children. For now these activities are a waste of time. Find them and eliminate them.

If you feel like you are constantly running out of time, take a closer look at what you do with your time and be realistic about how long things really take. Be critical, does this really need to be done in order to have a loving, happy, healthy, clean, fed and watered family?

Do you really need to iron baby clothes? Do you really need to fold vests and sleep suits? Is it essential to wash and change your babies' clothes every morning even though they've had a bath the previous evening and still smell fresh as daisies? Unless these activities add a great deal of pleasure and happiness to your life, why not eliminate them?

Whenever the girls both slept for an hour, I realised just how much there was to do and I simply didn't know where to start. My friend Charlotte had the solution, not a twin mum but a mum of three under four she found herself in a similar situation. Charlotte had a fortnightly jobs list on the kitchen wall, small non-daily jobs that she aimed to do on certain days of the week. Genius.

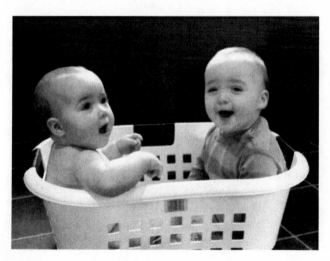

Amber and Ewan helping mummy Maria with the laundry.

This really worked for her and for me. It was obviously fine to do more and it wouldn't be a failure if things on the list were done the following day or not at all as time for a cuppa is just as important now and then, it was just a great tool in order to focus and make the most of time when available. One other great thing about this list is that you will only think of dreaded chores on the day you are planning to do them and simply not have to think about them for the rest of the week, which reduces stress.

Here are some other ideas:

• Household Olympics. Race yourself for example when doing chores you don't enjoy, set a stop watch and see how fast you can empty the dishwasher, hang up the washing or pick up toys. They don't really take that long. By the time you have thought about how to postpone them, you probably could have done most of it.

• Teach your children to place clothes in the washing basket, how to load or unload the washing machine, to take empty plates to the sink, they love it and it saves a few moments.

• Prepare breakfast, pre-pack bags, put shoes and clothes out in the evening if you can foresee time shortages the following morning.

• Touch it once. Don't just move it somewhere else, put it straight back where it belongs.

"*In terms of development, very young children [...] haven't mastered the ability to use logic and words to express their feelings, and they live their lives completely in the moment – which is why they will drop everything to squat down and fully absorb themselves in watching a ladybug crawl along the sidewalk, not caring one bit that they are late for their toddler music class. Logic, responsibilities, and time don't exist for them yet.*"

From the book: The Whole Brain Child,
by Dr. Daniel Siegel and Dr. Tina Payne Bryson,
Publisher: Bantam

RESET YOUR CLOCK

One thing I noticed about women who seemed to be in control was that they appeared to be moving much slower and finally I understood why, these clever ladies had adjusted their inner clocks, they had adjusted their expectations of how much time it takes a child to perform a simple task and they started moving accordingly, calm, slowly, effortlessly, preserving energy. EVERYTHING takes longer than it could take, that seems to be the law when having young children.

For example, getting a toddler to put his shoes on in adult-time and space takes a minute at the most and involves sitting down, putting shoes on, getting up again. In toddler time and space it might very well involve climbing into the rocket, firing up the engine and flying over to where the shoes live deep down the narrow hallway, landing on an unknown planet, climbing out the rocket and carefully putting on the shoes whilst continuously checking the functionality of the space suit, then taking off again and flying over to the front door avoiding several meteorites and flying pigs. This takes 5 minutes! Not one. And there is no need to shout as it can't be heard in space.

When dressing two little ones it also quite frequently happens that the first one has managed to take the socks off again by the time the second one is dressed. Getting in the car should only take a few minutes unless someone does a big poo and you have to start getting ready all over again. That's the way it is. So why rush and stress? You wouldn't put meat in a slow cooker and then shout at the machine for taking so much longer than your frying pan.

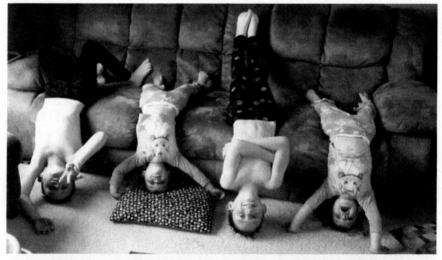

There is always time for routine-morning-stretches in Allison's household with her two sets of twins: brothers Elvis & Hank and their little sisters Betty and Roxi.

OPTIMISE ENERGY AND EFFORT

A routine is NOT what your babies are supposed to be doing;
it's what YOU are planning to be doing.

Create a routine

When I just had Jacob I didn't have a routine, I actually thought routines were pretty uncool. I didn't quite get what all the fuss was about and why some of my friends couldn't leave the house at certain times of the day or had to have dinner at exactly 5pm or else the world would come to an end. I just wanted to go with the flow, be flexible and get out as much as possible.

In the early months I breastfed every three hours and that was pretty much it. I didn't realise that this was actually my routine, everyone has a routine. It can be a strict regime which dictates when to drink a glass of water or it can be a simple rhythm such as every three hours feed and change the baby. As this worked fine with one baby I decided to have the same approach with my two babies the only thing I wanted to add was a bedtime ritual in order to have the evenings to ourselves and to send a clear message that night time wasn't playtime.

I was lucky that my girls were placed into a feeding routine during their first three weeks in hospital; I don't think my life would have been as organised had we left hospital after a few days. Apart from the feeding and nappy changing rhythm I didn't really have much of a plan for the first six months. I was breastfeeding my babies on demand during growth spurts and I was out and about a lot.

I did read about routines but I didn't really follow one. I didn't expect them to sleep through the night yet and got used to my little chunks of sleep. I was hoping that once they started solids they would sleep for longer periods at night.

So all was going really well, until I started weaning them - that's when I felt like losing any control I'd ever had. I had Jacob who was a fussy eater and always got in such a state when over hungry. Isla wasn't that much into food and had this fantasy of being hardwired to my boob, she pretty much always wanted a breastfeed the very minute I started spoon feeding Jess. During the first few weeks of weaning I cooked different foods for Jacob and the girls, later on they had the same just puréed for the babies. And it was ridiculous... I found myself cooking and feeding all day, one hungry, one not hungry or asleep and another over hungry demanding a different dinner or a glass of milk or buttered toast... and I simply didn't have enough arms to serve them all.

My hopes that the nights would be getting easier didn't come true either and I was exhausted and ready for some sleep. I needed a proper routine! Not just for them but also for myself, a structure to the day, a plan of when to do what, in order to get it all done. I consulted the different books I had bought or borrowed and tried sticking to some of them for a week or two but some just made it worse as our daily rhythm was just worlds away from the one suggested in the book, plus most didn't take the older sibling into consideration and the pre-school runs or even the fact that I was breastfeeding.

I felt myself getting stressed about establishing a routine and felt a bit like my children and I were a failure as we weren't able to fulfil the targets set by the books. Then I realised that this was completely defeating the point of having a routine in the first place. Yes, maybe I should have started earlier like many of the twin mums I met at twins club who chose a routine early on, stuck with it and were very happy with it. But I didn't and it was too late to change it.

I asked many twin mums and mums in general and concluded, there is no such thing as a "perfect" routine, there are only suitable ones and once you have found a suitable routine, it makes your life easier as your days become more predictable and you gain more control. One thing a routine definitely shouldn't be doing is causing stress whilst trying to establish it! Babies are unique, so are their parents, our personal circumstances are unique.

If you decide to try a book routine and it works: Great! If it doesn't work then it's not yours or your babies' failure – it's simply not suitable! Chuck the book in the corner and try another one or craft your own. Some books give a helpful insight into how much sleep a baby at a certain age requires or how often they should have a milk feed. This could be used as a starting point to tailor your own routine. Observing and keeping a log of natural sleep / eat / getting hungry / getting tired / play / alert patterns helps to develop your own routine.

Activities you should definitely include in your routine:
- tea break
- have something to eat yourself
- phone a friend
- sterilising
- any medications that need to be taken
- nap time for your children
- nap time for yourself
- (pre) school run if you have other children
- socialising

And any jobs you need to do or else they would stress you out.

For me this was "tidy up the kitchen in the evening" as I simply couldn't start the day in a messy kitchen and mornings really aren't the time to struggle.

The more I could see a pattern, the more I wanted a written routine. In the end I went for the Charlotte routine – never heard of it? I met my friend Charlotte at our local toddler group whilst our babies were still bumps; she is a nurse, a third time mum with two pre-school boys and a baby girl who was born four days after my girls. Charlotte is very sociable, just like me, and her day to day life and her kids sleep / feed patterns are actually quite similar to mine so I just copied her beautifully designed daily rhythm, tweaked her routine slightly to fit in two babies rather than one and also the fact that Isla had slightly different needs than her bigger sister Jess and it worked a treat! I think every twin mum should have a Charlotte in her life!

So I had my routine, my framework to reclaiming control over my life. Next thing was to write it down and to post in on the fridge (or kitchen wall, blackboard, mirror... it moved about a few times). This helped me to stay calm when things got a bit hectic and it also helped others, like my husband on his days off or anybody who gave me a helping hand, to know what was about to happen next. I still kept it quite flexible and tried to expect the unexpected, 4:30pm might be dinner time and food might be ready but one of the babies might not be cooperating. Call it food strike or maybe she's teething, maybe she simply hasn't read the schedule. Fact is, it's still dinner time for the willing one and you need to get her fed, whilst entertaining her twin and then try again a little later.

When things got hectic I used to focus just on the next milestone in my routine, and that way difficult days appeared broken up into manageable little chunks. Having a routine, a daily rhythm of what's going to happen next is not only reassuring for the parent but also or even more so for the children as being able to understand what comes next gives them a sense of security and stability.

It's important to remember that routines change with your babies, with their needs and their age and of course with personal circumstances. They tend to go out the window when someone gets sick or when going on holiday and it simply takes a bit of time to get back into it afterwards. Going for a walk or drive around nap time always seemed to do the trick, and having a bucket full of patience, of course.

Checklists and logs

Lists are a brilliant tool when things get a bit hectic and your brain is running at maximum capacity. They save you having to work out things over and over again, if it's an activity that repeats itself, write it down and next time you can just follow the list whilst concentrating on other things, such as a three year old asking five million questions about spiders and bugs whilst you need to get packed up for a day out. Examples are:

- packing list for a day out

- packing list for swimming

- telephone numbers of neighbours or other potential helpers who live nearby

- babysitter check list

- list with popular, easy kids meals

- master grocery list, items you always have to buy

- meal plan (could for example be fortnightly)

- cleaning plan

- medical log

The packing list for the day out, for example, could be stuck to your front door, that way anyone can help you with getting ready without the risk of forgetting any essentials.

Focus! One step at a time.

People often tell me: "I don't know how you do it" and I often reply "I don't know either". But one morning when taking my son to school I realised how I do it, I focus on the next step and that's it! I don't ever think how will I make it through the week or the next month or year? I only really concentrate on the next step. When things get a bit hectic I narrow my focus even further, I break down "getting ready to leave" into every single step involved such as putting on shoes, grabbing coats etc and concentrate just on that activity and nothing else. Focus! Keep control of the one thing you need to do right now. In order to do this, you need to plan ahead and stay in the moment and make it through the moment. Take a deep breath and take one step at a time!

Everything gets easier. My girls are 18 months old as I am writing these words and the morning school run wasn't stressful at all. The girls are now walking and into everything. I remember those early days with little sleep when the prospect of six weeks summer holidays with four months old twins and a three year old toddler seemed like a daunting task. But life is getting a lot easier, more predictable and so much fun!

Be over-prepared for big trips or holidays

We went to Spain when the girls were ten months old, I guess we could have just flushed the money for the trip down the loo, but at least we proved to ourselves that we could do it. The weather was rubbish, the girls just wanted to breastfeed all night long and when they woke up they screamed the place down in order to get back to what they believed was theirs to stay in their mouths all night. Rich pushed them round the hotel in the middle of the night just to get them to sleep for 20 minutes or so. And to top it all off we all caught a really nasty tummy bug and spent two days trapped in our hotel room being so ill that we actually had to phone a doctor. So the trip was rubbish – but our preparation had been meticulous.

We had practised and most importantly discussed all the different scenarios involved, like boarding the plane with three children and various pieces of hand luggage – one of us would kneel down and hold the girls whilst the other one would fold up the buggy, Jacob had to hold onto a strap attached to Rich's belt.

We also practised getting on the bus and collecting luggage from the luggage carousel. We talked about the girls' routine before the start of the holiday. On later trips we planned situations such as collecting the rental car, getting on the train (one parent first, the other last as you really don't want to leave any children on departing trains).

On planes and trains it's a good idea to have some cash in your pocket as it's tricky to get up just to dig for money. Same for nappies and wet wipes, muslin squares, bibs and some toys, we used to have a small bag for all these essentials and kept it by our feet. A change of clothes in the hand luggage is also a good idea.

Getting to the airport two hours before flight departure might be fine for adults travelling on their own, but with babies two hours might be cutting it a bit fine. On our next holiday we had a second bedroom and a fridge in the room, having milk and cereal for the mornings and evenings was a life saver.

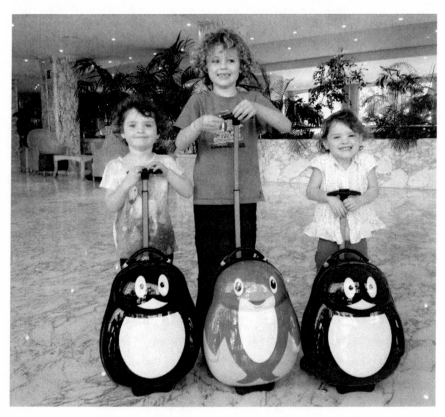

A few years later- now we're travel experts!

Clever Equipment

Another waste is using equipment that doesn't work. It just drives you mad, wastes time and takes up too much effort.

You don't need half of the things people tend to buy for babies, mine were perfectly happy without door bouncers and walkers, but then again there is equipment available that makes life just so much easier.

I believe the two most useful items, next to a feeding pillow (read the breastfeeding chapter for more info), are bath seats and a playpen. Here is why.

Bathing

At first they were so tiny, we bathed them in our bathroom sink, one at a time. We then moved onto a baby bath tub which we placed on the living room floor on a pile of hand towels. Again we bathed one first then the other. Then comes a time when you move onto the large bath tub and as your babies can't sit unassisted yet, you have to hold them. And that's fine and all I ever did with my singleton.

Ideally you prepare everything, lay the towels out etc. But then comes the day when you would like them to share the bath and you run out of hands to support them, unless you have a pair of helping hands. I used to bath our children before Rich got home and for quite a while my mother-in-law used to come over and help me with dinner and bath time. That was great! It was so much easier with two adults feeding and bathing three little children. But then there were times when I didn't have a helping hand.

I liked the idea of bathing all three children at the same time. I wanted to keep the girls in sync, I didn't want to leave one out and also because it's so cute having them all in the tub together.

The big bath madness started when they were able to sit unassisted, but even though the girls were capable of sitting, the crucial moment was when I had to get them out as I would have to take my eyes and hands off one of them in order to lift the other one out. A bath seat solved all my problems.

They would take it in turns to sit in the bath seat, this way I could take one out and dry her off next to the bathtub whilst keeping an eye on her brother and sister, knowing that she couldn't get out of the seat. Rachael from my twins club used a couple of reclined bath seats like the ones shown in the picture below which also looks like a great idea. My friend Charlotte used fabric bath seats. Second hand bath seats are always for sale somewhere.

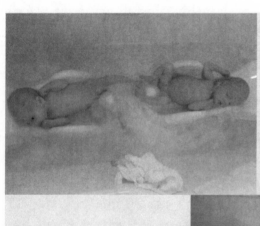

Mini Hattie and Bea in their baby bath seats.

Isla in the bath seat, Jess and Jacob roaming free.

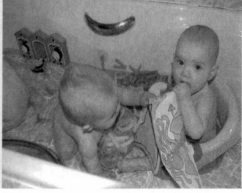

Playpens

Just being able to leave your children in a secure place for a moment whilst going to the loo is worth buying a playpen for. I had a big round playpen with a height adjustable floorboard. I knew my babies couldn't get anywhere when I left the room, my son wasn't allowed to climb into the playpen and therefore they were also safe from yummy looking small Lego pieces, from being accidentally hit by one of his rockets, racing cars or falling towers. Some of my friends with cats and dogs also used playpens to divide the different species in the house.

My kids all loved the playpen. When Jacob was a baby he pretty much learned how to walk by cruising round the inside of the playpen holding on to the side and the living room always seemed a tad tidier as the baby toys were all inside the playpen.

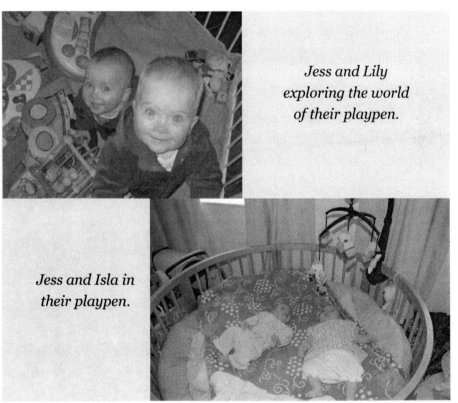

Jess and Lily exploring the world of their playpen.

Jess and Isla in their playpen.

MAKING THE MOST OF MATERIALS AND FACILITIES

I collected some more ideas on how to do more with less, so here is a fairly random list of waste avoiding ideas that I really had to include in this book.

- Do it like a childminder and only have a choice of toys out to keep them interested.

- Try and keep keys in one place, looking for a key is so frustrating.

- Have a box with any unwanted (children's) gifts, gifts you buy when you see them and a stash of birthday cards, that way you don't need to drag everyone out when you get a (last minute) birthday invitation.

- Make tidying up part of the game.

- Set up the breakfast table the evening before.

- Pack any lunch boxes and bags the evening before.

- Teach your children as early as possible to put their dirty washing in the basket or another designated place. This will pay off when they get older and start dressing and undressing themselves.

- Cook double batches and fill up your freezer with foods for your children and yourself.

- If your babies are in different size nappies, buy them from different brands as it saves lots of time not having to search for the size.

- Childproof your house early.

- At the bottom of the stairs, have a basket for anything that needs to be taken upstairs.

Glimpse into the future

Jess and Isla are nine months old. Routine all gone out the window again, girls cried so much last night, ended up feeding them at 4am, not what I had planned.

The Kitchen is a mess, laundry everywhere, Isla is crying upstairs overtired and wants to fall asleep with nipple in her mouth, my trousers are covered in milk and carrot, I haven't even looked in the mirror yet and it is already 2pm, now Jess starts crying. Jacob has been a little nightmare this morning and yesterday, must have a bug or something or he is simply trying to win the whinge world cup, pretty sure he will get the trophy!

I need a break, no more crying and whinging and talking to babies and toddlers. I feel like I am losing my mind … deep breath count to ten, think of the Maldives.

9:35am – **Jess and Isla are 14 months old.** Well sometimes just getting dressed seems to be "Mission Impossible". It's half past nine and only Isla is dressed and overtired as she has been up since 6am, Jacob (4) is glued to "Handy Manny" and has either gone deaf or maybe his mind is on another planet and he has just left his body in his PJs here on the lounge floor, you never know, after all he has electric arms and eyes. Jess is after my cuppa, I think she needs refreshments after the hard work of emptying out the nappy box and kindly spreading the formerly sorted size 3 and size 4 nappies pretty much all over the house. Maybe when Jacob returns to planet Earth I can convince him to play a 'fun' number game and sort them for me – in his PJs of course.

It's Monday morning, **Jess and Isla are 15 months old.** All kids slept through the night last night, the weather was so lovely yesterday that they just played in the garden all day long and all that fresh air must have helped. I give them dinner at 4:30 pm these days and they spoon and finger feed themselves even though they only have four teeth.

The mess when they eat is getting less too, which is great. Jacob, my four year old, loves that they are so much fun now. All three play hide and seek together, tickle one another, wash each other in the bath, go on the slide together and read books together. It's brilliant.

After dinner they all go for another play, walk, crawl around in the garden, at 5:30 / 6:00 pm they have a bath followed by story and milk and at about 6:30 pm I put Jess and Isla to bed, fully awake, in separate rooms as this currently just happens to work best for everyone. Jacob joins Jess in the upstairs bedroom at 7:15 pm and we hardly ever hear another peep from anyone and have the evening to ourselves. We spend the first hour getting the house back into a liveable shape and cook our own dinners.

Jess is the first one to wake up in the mornings, normally around 6am followed by Jacob. We go downstairs and play a bit in the lounge until we can hear little noises coming from the playroom where Isla sleeps. Big brother Jacob and Jess, who started walking a week ago, run into the playroom and they all have a laugh and a giggle and start playing instantly. Jess and Isla have some milk and then we all have breakfast at around 7:30am / 8am. They all eat the same now, toast and cereal, yoghurt and fruit and they feed themselves.

Jacob's friends (and their mothers of course) come to collect him for pre-school at 9:15am so we have plenty of time to play and to get washed, changed and dressed. By 9:30am the girlies are ready for their morning nap, I put them to bed awake, close the curtains and shut the door and they will then sleep until 11:30am / 12noon. Bliss! All these hard days of convincing them to sleep and working out a routine have certainly paid off! When I look back at how much harder it was only just six months ago then I wish I would have been able to take a quick glance into the future and see how much easier it will get. This was YOUR glance into the future!

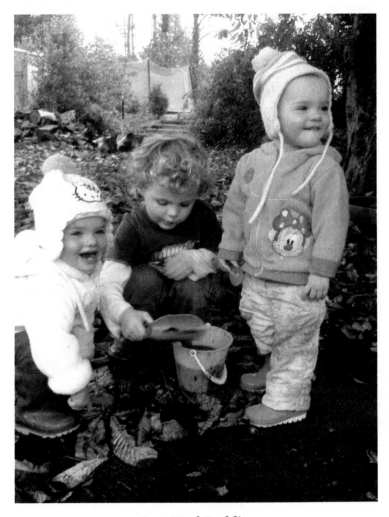

Best Mud Buddies
Jess, Jacob and Isla.

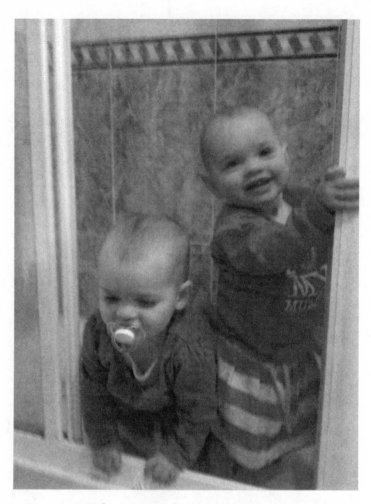

Did you say "shower", mummy?

{CHAPTER 7}

HEALTHY SELF EXPECTATIONS

Being a mum is the best paid job in the world
as it's paid in 100% true love and cuddles .

Some days it's late in the afternoon and I haven't even had lunch, or it's the evening and I haven't looked in the mirror once. It just happens, I keep forgetting about myself. Whilst I was breastfeeding I made sure to eat and drink enough but once the girls went onto solids and started to be on the move, I just seemed too busy looking after them to look after myself. Whenever I make an effort to wear something nice I end up with a selection of slobber, milk, carrot or chocolate stains. I am forever eating the kids leftovers (waste not, want not), I do own jewellery and I am aware of how to use mascara, I just keep forgetting to use either.

I sometimes catch myself thinking "I just want my old life back" and a second later it makes me smile as this is probably the most ridiculous idea ever, how can I possibly get my life before children back now that I've had children? These little people have changed everything, my daily life, my job, my priorities, my hopes and fears, and not to forget my boobs and bum.

Yes of course, there are a lot of things I can do again after pregnancy or breastfeeding. Those two babies might no longer be doing somersaults in my womb, I can go for a run, indulge in sushi or drink way too much wine, but I can't get my old life back. That's a fact. I don't want it back but I believe it's still important to get back into aspects of 'life before children' thought. May that be a certain body shape, hobbies or getting back into the old job, just to name a few. It's all about finding a way to not lose yourself in being a mum alone and at the same time feeling like a good mum. I know I am a good mother, but sometimes I feel like I am failing to achieve all the things I would love to achieve, such as teaching my twins how to count, do puzzles and read as much as I did with my singleton.

I think in one way or another being a twin mum comes with having unrealistic self expectations. May this be from seeing and reading about super mums, super slim famous mums or the perfectly groomed, top career mum across the road.

You set yourself up to fail if you have too high expectations and failure doesn't feel good. You don't enjoy your job if you think you're not good at it and this job here is all about enjoying yourself and your family. The key is to have realistic expectations and not to give yourself and your own needs up completely.

Whenever I speak to other mums, twin mums or pregnant ladies there appear to be the same topics:

- Trying to be the perfect mum

- Getting back into shape

- Stay-at-home mum

- Silly guilt

- Individuality

- Zero Power days

- If you do hit rock-bottom

"Oh hello, I am looking for the perfect mum, have you seen her?"

"Yes sure, she is just over there feeding her Unicorns."

TRYING (NOT) TO BE THE PERFECT MUM

I read this lovely saying somewhere: "There is no way to be a perfect mother, but a million ways to be a good one."

What's perfection anyway? I checked the dictionary and the definition of perfect is: "The condition, state, or quality of being free or as free as possible from all flaws or defects." That sounds really boring and uninspiring. Who judges anyway? In the world of retail shopping, it's the customers judging the quality of a product, service, store or brand, if they are happy, spending their money and returning for more, then it's a great business.

So when it comes to mums' business who better to be the judges than the children (we don't tell them that though as it leaves too much room for blackmail). I asked some children: "Why is your mum a good mum?"

Here are their answers:

- She makes pancakes, draws dinosaurs and likes Scooby Doo. (Finn, 5)

- She is beautiful and gives me lots of kisses. (Joseph, 5)

- She makes good dinners, spends all the time with us, best in the world at cooking and she has lovely hair! (Jo, 3)

- Because she gives me sweets. (Luisa, 4)

- Because her cuddles are nice! (Lina, 3)

- She bakes cakes and she carves pumpkins with me. (Josh, 5)

Now, that's more like it, anyone surprised they didn't mention a tidy kitchen, a clean car or nicely folded or even ironed laundry? Baking was mentioned, and yes I like the idea of baking with my three young children, I also like the idea of them baking with granny instead. And I feel the same for crafting. I love it if they do craft at toddler groups, pre-school and now and again at home but there is only so much glitter glue I can handle in a month and it's certainly not a regular activity in our house at the moment. But no doubt it will be, once paint and glue actually end up on paper rather than in their mouths and hair.

And now to sort out a few more misconceptions, you're not a bad mother when you let your children watch television now and then. A study by the BabyCentreUK found that nine out of ten mums do occupy their children for a while. 71% of parents admitted to using little white lies now and again (the ice cream van plays music when it's run out of ice cream, daddy can't hear you when he is in the office, this teddy bear has super powers and will look after you whilst you sleep, there is no chicken in chicken nuggets, sorry darling but the softplay area is closed today because a little boy did a big poo in the ballpool and now they need to wash all the balls). The US magazine Parenting found that 23% of mums crave alone time sometimes, away from the children.

GETTING BACK INTO SHAPE

When I started breastfeeding the weight just fell off – despite my daily intake of four chocolate bars, fetched from the hospital vending machine at pretty much any time of the day. It was brilliant. I was also losing all the water my body had stored, my elephant feet had disappeared and all in all I lost 22kg in the first 3 weeks after giving birth, this obviously includes two babies and all the gear that came with them. I'd be back into my pre pregnancy clothes in no time! Wishful thinking!

The weight loss stopped there. I continued to be very hungry, ravenous at times, which was fine as I wanted to give my daughters the best breast milk they could get and whenever I felt like eating chocolate or cheese I simply did, as I believe it's the body's way to tell you what ingredients it needs right now to create some yummy milk for the offspring. I walked a lot with the double buggy and felt quite fit. I was really enthusiastic about going to exercise classes but leaving two babies in the crèche and then being called out half way through the class in order to change a nappy or two turned out to be a rather expensive and not very successful experience. Some evenings I managed to source enough energy to go to Zumba, for a run or a swim, but it certainly wasn't enough to get back into the shape I wanted to be in.

When I stopped breastfeeding I tried sticking to a low carbohydrate diet but soon realised that my busy life with three little children required a lot of energy and therefore screams for carbohydrates. So what to do? What diet to try next?

And then I read about the findings of Albert Einstein College of Medicine in New York who found, that when starved of food, brain cells actually start eating one another. No way would I sacrifice brain cells for a smaller dress size. I had only just recovered from pregnancy-brain-freeze and was enjoying being able to accurately calculate my five year olds year one sums. So all further diet plans were cancelled. The other issue was that I still wasn't getting much sleep.

SLEEP has an impact on weight loss. When you're tired you need quick energy and might opt for foods high in sugar or fat and you generally have less energy for additional exercise. Several studies have shown a link between little sleep and little success at losing weight, some studies conclude that sleep deprived woman have more of the hormone that tells us to eat and less of the hormone that signals us to stop eating. Other studies say that insufficient sleep leads to a higher release of stress hormones which in turn can stimulate hunger. Others link it to less growth hormones being released, higher blood glucose levels and therefore higher fat storage. Whatever the causes, it appears there really is a link and if you're getting little sleep and trying to lose weight at the same time you might feel like you're fighting a losing battle – and you are! Once I came to realise this, I just postponed my plan to get back into shape. I eventually had more energy to do sports and I was in the right frame of mind to concentrate on my own dinners without having to fight yet another battle. Alternatively you could just decide to be happy the way you are and concentrate on other things!

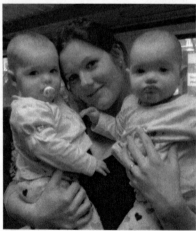

My daily workout.

"So what do you do for work?"
"I am having a career break."

STAY AT HOME MUM / HOMEMAKER

I take my hat off to those returning to work once their maternity leave is up. Working mums out there, doing incredible jobs despite sleep deprivation. Ingrid, the oncology nurse, who comes home to baby twin boys Jack and Oliver; Carrie the primary school teacher who marks homework once she's put her four young children to bed – you ladies are amazing!

For us, childcare was simply not available. For some of my friends the cost of childcare would have outweighed their earnings. So we became stay at home mums (SAHM) / house wives / homemakers for the first few years of our twins' lives. Which is a privilege, of course, but I did long to return to work, if just for a break. The trick to enjoying my new job as SAHM was to really embrace it.

Let me tell you a little story from when my twins were ten months old: Yesterday was great, I felt like super mum! Got up at half past six, successfully fed all three kids breakfast without any drama, packed a lunchbox for Jacob, walked (!) to pre-school, all dressed properly (!) and got there on time (!), went for breakfast with some friends, no drama lunch for the girls, collected Jacob in time, took them all to the library and had a fun time there, did a little food shop, went home and gave the children their dinner (again no drama), bathed them all on my own and put them all to bed on my own, even managed to make a hot water bottle for Jacob and told him two stories! Oh... and cooked dinner for Rich. I am officially Super Twin Mum of Three! So pleased with myself was I, I had to shout it out to the world via social network status, lots of praise and happiness from other mums and female friends and one comment by a male university mate: "Isn't that what is expected from a stay at home mum / house wife?"

And that brings super twin mum straight down to earth, flight's over. It's been bugging me all morning.

My reply was: "If you mean "stay at home mum" as in HR Manager, Judge, Event Manager, Teacher, 5* Chef, Race Driver, Fortune Teller also in charge of acquisition and disposal, health care and mental well being, working hours 24/7 then yes! That's what is expected."

I should have just ignored his comment as I don't have to justify anything, and yet I do, but I guess stay-at-home mums get this occasionally, maybe from their own partners, sneaky little remarks that might make you feel 'less worthy', just a mum, not an achievement to get pregnant and pop out children, woman do it all the time all over the world...

So doesn't that indicate that being a mum is THE MOST popular job in the WORLD, and as this job comes in so many variations, with so many different job descriptions, it might very well be the hardest job in the world – as the outcome is of such major importance!

Maybe anybody can be a mum, but are they all great, loving mums who raise healthy, happy, confident people? That's where the challenge lies, just like with any important job! I can do the prime minister's job, I can do my mate's consultancy job, I can also start tomorrow and do my husbands job but will I be as good as these people? Will I get it right? Probably not!

And if they did my job, would they be as great as I am, would they get it right?

Definitely not!

It's the outcome that matters - your children, nothing else! If you feel someone is belittling you for being a mum just ask yourself what is the outcome of this person's daily job and then take a look at what you are doing, look at your beautiful children and there you have it, you are onto a winner here.

And if it helps, try and put a value to your job. How much would a childminder or your local nursery charge 24/7 for two babies, plus meals? And don't forget to add at least an extra 20% for the hours between 6pm and 6am.

IT'S ALL BABY TALK NOW – TIME TO BE SILLY!

"He says all us mums ever talk about is babies..." Yes of course, that's what professionals do when they meet for working lunch, they talk about work and their achievements. My husband runs a retail business and when he meets up for dinner with a supplier all they talk about is based around products and pricing, that's just what us mums do, discuss the latest gadgets, prices and tricks of the trade. When I meet my colleagues (other mums) we talk about routines, time saving strategies, efficient use of wet wipes (yes there is such thing – I only need two where my other half needs half a pack) and so much more exciting stuff! And when the babies were little, there honestly wasn't much time or space for anything other than baby business and anyone asking me what I had been doing all day, last week or even last month my answer would have been baby talk. And that's the way it is, no point complaining about it, time to embrace it! If you're spending so much time with your children, why not behave like one of them now and then, be totally silly, talk nonsense, pretend you speak cat language, pretend you have wobbly legs, you can't stop shaking your hair or you need to lick your kids' ears and pretend you want to eat their feet. They will LOVE it! It's great for distraction and tantrum avoidance too.

SILLY GUILT

Talk to any mum with more than one child and I bet you they've felt what I call "silly guilt". It's the feeling that you are not giving enough attention or spending enough individual time with one of your children, either one of your babies or in many cases the older sibling when a baby or two arrive. Sometimes one baby needs more attention than the other, for example this could be because feeding takes longer or maybe they need special therapy or medicines. Having spoken to mums with special needs children it appears that the healthier twin grows to be the best helper they could ask for, they tend to comfort their twin and at the same time help their twin to develop. Maybe the thing to remember here is that your children simply don't know any differently. When you have one child who is more demanding than the other, then it might be an option to get a babysitter or friend to occupy the one fussing whilst you enjoy some quality time with the other.

Older siblings get less attention than before simply because it takes time to feed, change and dress two babies. I remember one morning when I was getting my girls ready and Jacob was sat on the couch and asked me if I used to dress him and cuddle him so much. Pang! Silly Guilt! From that day on I started telling the girls everything about their big brother whilst changing or dressing them, about how he loves his teddy Pandi and what his friends are called and why I love him so much, and he used to sit next to us and laugh his head off. I also started helping him to put his clothes on, even though he had been doing it unassisted for ages, it just shows him that I love him just as much as his baby sisters.

Sometimes I get to the end of the day and feel like I haven't given anyone any individual attention, but it's silly really, as I have. Every sentence you just address to one of them, every shoe you put on their feet, every spoon you feed one and look them in the eyes and say their name and not to forget every toilet visit. It's all individual attention.

INDIVIDUALITY

When having twins, Individuality is a big talking point. I went to a TAMBA workshop where we discussed individuality and established that the aim was "to raise a mature dependent individual who is a multiple" (rather than closely coupled or extreme individual). This goes beyond the dress code, it's about how to spend individual time with just one of them and to give them undivided attention, how to nurture their different personalities, how to praise one without the other one feeling left out and having their own possessions at the same time as being able to share with one another.

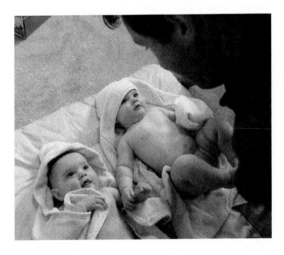

Daddy Rich teaching Isla and Jess their names whilst towelling them down after a bath.

Here are a few ideas I picked up during the workshop:

• Every sentence addressed to one child only, including their name is 1:1 time.

• Nappy changing is great 1:1 time – and it easily adds up!

• Don't label them, the "smart" one etc.

• When it was their first birthday I got upset because they got joint cards and presents. I wanted friends and family to acknowledge they were individuals. Then I realised I had send out a joint birthday invite.

• When one achieves something, celebrate with the other.

• Mine have special toys they don't need to share.

• Don't try to be fair all the time; it will even out over the years anyway.

• Praise achievement and praise the other one's effort.

• Cut out the comparison.

• It is okay to let your kids play on their own for a while, it teaches them to be independent and creative.

ZERO POWER DAYS

Some days not all the management skills and checklists in the world can change the fact that I am too shattered to do anything. I just feel like doing nothing. And that's fine! Those days I call Zero Power days and yesterday was one. I woke up in the morning with absolutely zero power, totally washed out. You might experience these days, one day you feel like on top of the world, your head is full of ideas how to sort the wardrobe, weaning recipes and all that exciting stuff that comes with being a new mum, and the next day you can hardly face getting dressed or even getting the kids dressed. And you know what? It doesn't matter as tomorrow is another day.

I have come to realise that if you try too hard on these days, you will only get stressed and run down and you won't get anything done anyway. Your babies and other children will feel that you're stressed too and will make it extra challenging. Much better to accept these days as Zero Power Days and only aim to achieve the bare essentials: having fed and watered children at the end of the day. It's not going to hurt your babies if they stay in their sleepwear all day and don't have a bath. Stick to the essentials such as nappy changing and feeding and of course lots and lots of cuddling! Always have the buggy and some clothes ready to go for a walk, great for zero power days! A few blankets for the babies is all you need, leave the change bag untouched, just get out and clear your head! So, yesterday I didn't do anything but make it through the day, my only other achievement was to send my husband a text warning him that it's been a zero power day so he got us a take away and ignored the mess at home. I had an early night and today really is another day and I feel much better.

IF YOU DO HIT ROCK BOTTOM

Having the occasional Zero Power Day and having moments or even days when you feel it's all too much are part of the first years with twins or even just one baby. If you find that these moments are taking over and you don't really enjoy your twins, yourself, if you can't find the power to eat properly, laugh or you don't ever feel like leaving the house anymore, then you might suffer from postnatal depression, which is more common for mothers of multiples.

If you do hit rock bottom remember that you are not a bad mother and you DO love your children, it's just that a lot of factors have contributed to you feeling the way you do right now. Did you feel sick during the first trimester? I did. But I wasn't sick of being pregnant; it was the cocktail of chemicals in my body. Some tricks eased the sickness and luckily it just disappeared. PND is also affected by changes in your body that are out of your control but it won't just disappear like the morning sickness did. It's nothing to feel ashamed of and the silly thing is that once you acknowledge what's happening you will feel a little better already.

Talk to a health professional, midwife or general practitioner or get your partner, or a friend or relative to make an appointment for you. If you believe you don't need medical help then at least talk to another mum, your own mum or even a random woman on the street, chances are she has experienced it herself.

Did you know that PND isn't always treated with medication? Recent research has proven that psychological and social therapies are also very effective. So don't hold back talking to a professional just because you want to avoid talking any medication.

One big problem with PND is that once you are depressed you

tend to feel too low to do something about it. You might just feel shattered, empty, disinterested and you might not want to phone your friends or family, you don't want anything. Some mums described that they physically couldn't do anything, not even pick up the phone. So why not discuss this issue with some close friends whilst you are feeling great. Make them aware of it and ask them to check on you if they haven't heard from you in a while. And when they do, months later, you might just be snowed under a pile of washing and dirty nappies but over the moon that your babies are now saying "mummy" or you might be telling your friend that you are feeling a bit low and she will just know what's going on.

Visit www.tamba.org.uk for a valuable guide on PND and to watch related videos. Registration is free and available to all.

I sometimes imagine depressive thoughts to be nasty little trolls, who try to make you believe that you are not happy, not coping, some even go as far as to tell you that you don't love your children or yourself.

Don't believe them!

They feast on your bodily changes, on your lack of sleep, on isolation and too little fresh air. They hate it if you meet a friend or neighbour for some food and a walk in the sun or the rain. They hate if you nap in the daytime and the thing they hate the most is when you talk about them.

LIFE IS GREAT!

I think sometimes we just forget how great life is – because it is unpredictable, exciting, full of challenges and surprises, "a box of chocolates", and "you never know what's around the corner". If it wasn't for all the above – life would be boring.

You don't mop the floors during your own party; you enjoy those who are there to celebrate with you! Don't stress about what you haven't achieved, if the reason for living is the survival of the species as some claim, then you have already succeeded and everything else is just party clutter!

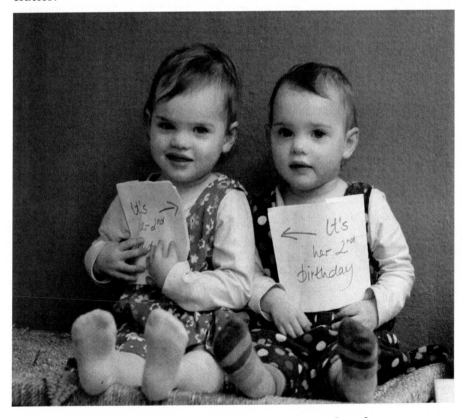

How time flies, my little girls are two already.

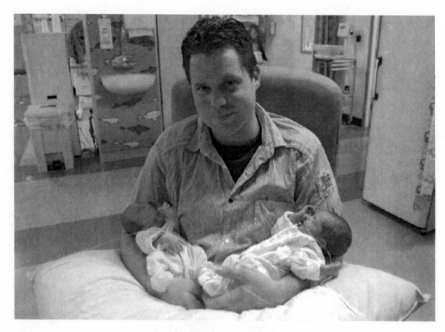

*A new twin-dad is born; Rich with Isla and
Jess in neonatal care.*

{CHAPTER 8}

REALISTIC RELATIONSHIP EXPECTATIONS

Having babies means you now have permission to cuddle someone other than your partner and it turns out the little ones cuddle much better and they are just so cute - it's really easy to forget to cuddle your older one too.

When I was pregnant I read an article in an American magazine claiming that marriages of twin parents are much more likely to end in divorce. Slightly upset and at the same time intrigued I decided to look into proper divorce statistics. I never got around to doing it though, as I was way too busy looking after my own relationship.

One evening when Jess and Isla were 18 months or so, Rich and I were sat in our local pub and overheard a (very loud and tipsy) woman telling (everyone) how her marriage broke up when their baby was six months old and they just stopped talking to one another as they didn't agree with certain aspects of parenting and all I could think was how sad it was that they hadn't managed to resolve their problems.

My best friend frequently phones me to announce that she's had enough of her partner and to be completely honest I was quite fed up at times and I am sure my husband was too. I have met numerous mums who would have sold their partners for a penny on eBay during the first months after having a baby or two.

I know there are a million reasons why relationships end, why feelings change and I certainly don't want to tell anyone to stay together "because of the children". But sometimes I think that if all arguments are solely due to baby-business, and there's no cheating or beating going on – why not put the whole breaking up business on hold until life gets a little bit easier? Until you have eliminated the possibility that you might just argue over the colour of blue. Remember that certain parenting issues will no longer be an issue once your children get a little older. If you give up on your relationship when your babies are little, you might miss out on something that could have been great a year down the line.

Rich keeps telling me a story about this gold miner who invested all his money into this massive dig, and he dug and dug and dug and then he realised he only had a little bit of money left and decided not to invest anymore. He kept the last few pennies in his wallet and walked away from the dig. He sold all his equipment and the rights to dig and within a matter of days, just another foot from where he had given up digging – his buyer found the biggest gold reserve seen to date. I have no idea how much of this story is true and how much of it is my husband's creative input – the point is however that relationships are put to the test and are under a lot of pressure when little people arrive, but once you have found your way and your family starts to play as a team, you are about to find gold, but it might be hard work at times.

When you add a baby or two to your little family, the dynamics change completely. Before it was just you and your partner, it was all about exclusivity and intimacy – you only cuddled and kissed one another, you only loved one another. Maybe there were mortgages and bills that needed paying – these were your only shared responsibility. Your bed used to be the place where you would not just sleep and your evenings you'd spend doing what you enjoy doing together, maybe snuggled up on the couch watching completely pointless stuff on television. Then these little people come along, and you love them so much, maybe more than your partner? Certainly in a totally different way! You spend hours cuddling, rocking and stroking your babies, not your partner. The dynamics have changed completely, intimacy is reduced, time spent together is filled with new tasks, new responsibilities. Some couples adjust to this just fine; others struggle and mourn the loss of their relationship. Well, fact is, you can't get back what you had as it's changed – YOU have changed it! It's time you not only get used to your new babies but also to get used to being with a partner who has multiples and who still needs cuddles and closeness and communication.

It's not a competition between the two of you – it's a team effort. Your family, your house, the bills that need paying – it's like one big project and you need to work as a team in order to be successful and happy. The one going out to work and bringing in the money shouldn't carry the burden of being financially responsible for the family, it's a shared "burden", you have chosen one of your team to go out and earn a living whilst the other takes on looking after the children. But it's just not that simple in real life, when you're tired and fed up and communication is at a minimum level. Communication and physical closeness suffer first; actively making an effort to improve both will help any relationship. So let's talk about TALK and TOUCH.

A little MORE conversation
and a little MORE action.

TALK AKA COMMUNICATION

"My partner doesn't have a clue what I do all day." If, in your relationship, dad has a fulltime job and you are the one spending all day with your babies, how can he possibly have an idea what you do? He is not the one doing it. It works both ways; you also don't know what he does all day or how often he thinks about you and your children, how the nightly interruptions affect him even though he might not be the one having to get up at night, how much he hates to miss out on so many things or how much of an outsider he feels during the first minutes of coming home to the madhouse and the gang ruling in it.

A mum's common complaint is that dad doesn't have a clue what she actually does and this offers plenty of material for evening- filling, totally pointless arguments. Other all time favourites include: "You didn't wind her properly", "You didn't put that nappy on properly" or "It's you who woke them". But those arguments are no reason to break up or leave one another!

But a father underestimating what mothers do all day is a big topic. I came across a joke the other day and it just fits so well into this chapter:

A man came home from work and found his three children outside, one of them wearing nothing but a woolly hat, the other two in pyjamas, playing in the mud, the house was totally trashed, there was food all over the place, paint spread across the floors, a little poo on the bathroom floor, toothpaste on the windows and the DVD collection in the bathtub. He ran upstairs and found his wife in bed reading a book. "What the heck happened here?"

She replied: "You know how sometimes you come home and ask me what I do all day? Well, today I didn't do it."

Very stereotypical and a tad sexist but it really made me laugh! And whilst we're at it, here's a naughty thought I had the other day: If men had babies we'd all be born via c-section (emergency c-section if labour accidentally starts before elective section date) and they would spend the last five weeks of the pregnancy on gas and air and Playstation! Only joking ... seriously! But all jokes aside, working dads might escape a lot of the twin chaos but twins still have a major impact on their lives and as a mum we might not always be able to see how much dad really does and how much effect there is on his working life. My husband once complained that nobody ever asked how he was coping, just how I was. Same goes for the praise, so far nobody has told him what an amazing twin dad he is but apparently I am bathing in praise (nice to know).

Tamba have published a leaflet about family relationships in families with multiples. It's an interesting read and can be downloaded from their website. I would like to quote one section, which lists some possible effects of having multiples on fathers:

- Fathers of twins are more likely to be involved [...] but may also lack the confidence in their ability to do so.

- They may feel isolated by the close relationship of the mother and multiple group.

- Fathers of multiples may feel additional pressure to help at home and cope with the pressure at work. The additional financial burden on the family may well increase that pressure.

And when it comes to the popular topic of what mums do all day: some men just get it; others don't see what's involved and need to be told or shown. An all time favourite is to throw him in at the deep

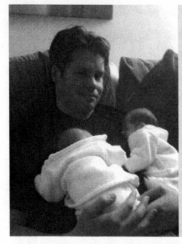

*Sleep deprived
daddy Rich.*

end, leave him in charge and leg it for a day or at least a morning.

If you want him to help when he gets back from work and you happen to be with someone who is a famous mind reader – congratulations, you're sorted. If you are not with a mind reader you will have to resort to actually telling your partner what would be helpful, how and when to do it! A routine on the fridge is a great tool.

My husband told me once, that when he comes home from work he usually parks the car next to our house and then stays in the car for another couple of minutes just to get mentally prepared for whatever is awaiting him indoors. "Come on, it's not that bad" I said. And he explained that the challenge is that he simply doesn't know what's happened throughout the day, have they slept a lot or will they go to bed alright? Has anyone been sick today? Is twin-mum in a bearable mood? He explained how he mentally files away his day at work whilst sat in the car and it wasn't until I went back to work for a couple of days and he had the kids that I actually started to understand. Suddenly it was me coming home to the big unknown. I was sad that I had missed out on a whole day with my children and at the same time I was quite tired from a busy day at work and wanted nothing more than to chill with my other half and do what adults do (talk and watch television that is).

We didn't really fall out much; I guess we got it out of our system when we had our first born. But sometimes it was challenging, and it was mostly during the night when we started arguing, comments like "you didn't wind her properly", "your baby woke mine" etc just don't really help the situation, and all you want and need at night is sleep! If you haven't read the chapter SLEEP yet, don't forget to do so as sleep is a cure to many a relationship issue. We decided to discuss any sleep arrangements in the daytime and not to fall out with one another in the middle of the night. During times of heavily interrupted nights we would sleep in separate beds just to get some much needed shut eye. You don't have to sleep in the same bed to be close to one another, you can cuddle on the couch instead – which takes us to the next important ingredient of a healthy relationship.

TOUCH AKA PHYSICAL CLOSENESS

This isn't (just) about sex; it's about holding hands, hugging and cuddling more than anything else. Having spent all day cuddling cute little babies or sweet little kiddies, it's easy to forget to cuddle one another. For many new parents there often isn't much energy, time or opportunity left at the end of the day to be intimate. Once a few months without much physical contact have passed, it might just become a habit not to touch one another and therefore much more of a challenge to actually get it going again.

During one of my interviews for this book, a mother of twins told me about her *zero libido situation*, and how it just doesn't happen when you've battled to get the kids to bed, tidy the mess and make some food and then realise you only have 20 minutes left before you ought to go to bed and there simply isn't much electricity left to get them going. Another lady described how she and her partner had been having scheduled sex for years simply in order to conceive the two reasons why they were now not having any romance at all.

Having a baby has the potential to put any relationship to the test, having two or more babies even more so. But Romance isn't dead. Romance just has been put in the cupboard and is patiently waiting to be released when the babies make some space for it. Some couples climb Mount Everest together, which takes 4-10 days and nights, involves sleeping in a tent in extreme temperatures and is extremely hard work, but you wouldn't do that and then complain half way up the mountain that romance is dead and search for a cosy restaurant and a cinema. You probably wouldn't hold hands during the climb but you might give each other a hand on the way up, help the other and get through it together. Romance can come out of the cupboard when you're back home and looking at the pictures.

I believe it can quickly become a habit not to touch one another, and then it's difficult to go from zero to 100% passion. But just like it has become a habit not to hug and kiss, it's a habit you can rebuild. You could even have some fun with it and one week always hold hands whilst watching a movie, or one proper kiss every day at 7 pm or a backrub on Tuesdays... anything really to get back in touch with one another.

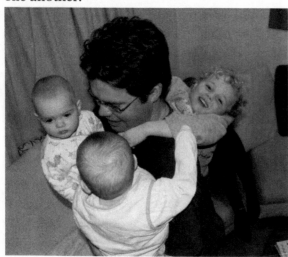

Home from work-hugs.

I asked other twin mums what their advice would be, here it is:

*"In all the mayhem, madness, chaos and mess, always
make time for each other! Daniel and I love our 'date
nights' and although they are very few and far between,
when we go out it makes everything worth while! Having
a baby, or two, or three is enough to take its toll on any
relationship, but finding that time together is a reminder
of what you have been through together and the amazing
little people
you now share it with."*
Gemma, mum to Sophie and Heidi, Barrett

*Working as a team has been vital to making it work for
our family. I know I couldn't do it without Pete's strong
support. At times it all feels so overwhelming. We keep
each other going and stronger.*
Lindy, mum to Albert, Arthur & Eddie

*"I think that I am very lucky because before the boys were
born we agreed that I would feed the babies, and he would
feed and water me, when you're breastfeeding it's hungry
and thirsty work and time consuming! Once he went out
of an evening and there wasn't anything to eat at home
so he'd offered to get fish and chips on his way back, but
he was two hours late and when he got home I was really
tearful and hungry. After that he started cooking stews
that would last a few days so there was always something
which could keep the wolf from the door! Looking back, I*

realise I have a very good thoughtful husband. I can get a little wobbly when I'm tired and I REALLY appreciated a little positive feedback regularly, you know stuff like "you're doing a great job" and 'I'm proud of you' and I think he has appreciated that sort of thing too, I regularly make a point of telling him I think he's a good dad (he is). Oh, and finally, both of us have a bit of our own space regularly, he goes climbing once a week or goes out with his buddies, and if ever I want to go out, he's happy to have the boys on his own. I haven't done it that much, but it's fun when I do."

Chloe, mum to Hector and Felix

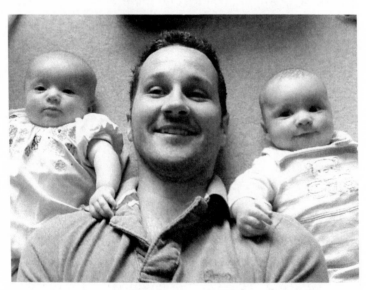

Hands-on daddy Rob with Ellie and Brad.

50 SHADES OF HAVING TWINS

Foreplay consists of picking up various Duplo bricks, cars and dinosaurs in order to clear a narrow path to the bed, remove a football, unused nappies and a choice of socks from the actual bed.

You lie down, get up again to carefully close the door and creep back to the bed cautiously avoiding the squeaky floorboards you really should have sorted before you put the carpet down.

"Shall we get the handcuffs out darling?"

"Sorry honey, the kids used them to arrest the cat and they managed to lose the key."

"What did they arrest the poor cat for?"

"Oh, just some petty-crime."

"Well, let me whip you a bit darling."

"Oh, can we do that another day, honey, Christian and Anna are due a feed in 15 minutes."

"A few clamps maybe?" "Naaaa..."

"Straight to the point then, not even foreplay?"

"Excellent idea darling, that's perfect."

Sounds like a *bestseller* to me!

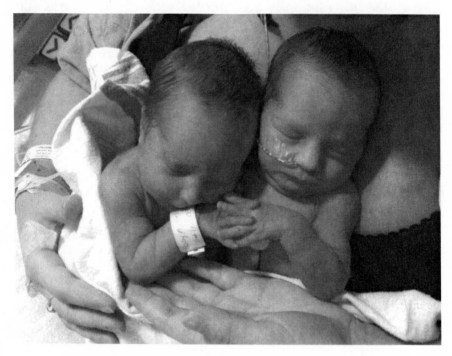

Katy enjoying a cuddle with her newborn twins
Stella and Sophie in neonatal care.

CHAPTER 9

THE BIRTH AND A STAY IN THE NEONATAL CARE UNIT

*"Birth plans are a silly thing; I have yet to meet a woman
where the birth went to plan. You start life as a mum
with a failed plan; a totally avoidable failure."*
Theresa, Mental Health Nurse

Every mother has a story to tell as every pregnancy and every birth is different, full of expectations, surprises, worries and pure wonder. Having two babies growing inside your body and giving birth to them is an incredible event and you spend weeks in eager anticipation of what the birth will be like and at how many weeks you will be delivering.

In my case, the answers to my questions kept changing on a fortnightly basis, depending on Isla's growth. I was told early on that the consultants recommend a delivery via c-section as my girls were sharing the placenta. I was so upset when I first heard of the c-section. I must have been driving my friends and family round the bend with all my talk about how I'd be delivering these babies naturally, with no pain relieve what so ever, just like I did with Jacob. It soon became evident, that I wouldn't and the closer I got to the delivery date, the more happy I was to have a c-section. I was so shattered by the end of the pregnancy that I was quite happy to skip labour. And then suddenly I was told that we'd have to bring the delivery date forward as Isla wasn't doing well. There was barely any time to contemplate what had actually happened. All of a sudden the pregnancy was over and done with and there I was, with two babies and my hands full. It's a bit like running to catch the train to twinland - the things you do to catch that train are mind blowing. You get a lift from a superhero, you ride your final mile on the back of a unicorn across some pretty scary moors, you then jump onto the train just as it is departing and holding on with just one finger you pull yourself onto the train seconds before entering a tunnel at 250 miles per hour. But there is no time to sit down and appreciate that you made it and how incredibly lucky you were to have made it. There is just too much happening right from the arrival in twinland. You keep taking more and more photos but you barely ever have the time to look at them. But that's the way it is. It's not about how you get there; it's about being there.

We all love birth stories, we even watch them on television. I have collected a few birth stories and am including them in this chapter. Some of the babies I will be telling you about were born very early and their birth stories are unusual, but they are also uplifting. I feel they have the potential to help someone who finds themselves in a similar situation. The last story is one where everything went very smooth and something quite funny happened.

Many twins are born a little earlier than expected; a twin pregnancy tends to be shorter for various reasons. There is a fair chance of a newborn twin spending some time in the neonatal care unit ((NNU), also called Special Care Baby Unit (SCBU) and I think every expectant twin parent should get some idea about what a stay in neonatal care involves. I came across so many amazing tiny, little people who started life earlier than expected and with parents who were so worried and shattered. And now, a couple of years later, these children are all doing incredibly well.

This chapter wasn't written with the intention to scare anyone, but to reassure. To help with being mentally prepared for what might lie ahead, even if never needed.

At the end of the chapter, you find my own birth and NNU diary. I kept a daily diary as I found it all to be such a rollercoaster of emotions. Trying to establish breastfeeding, expressing, having two babies in incubators and a toddler at home, recovering from a c-section and trying to get some sleep – it was quite a challenge.

Rest, sleep and eat whilst in neonatal care.
It's the calm before the storm!

A STAY IN NEONATAL CARE

When I was pregnant a lady at twins club told me how she and her hubby went to the pub for a meal when her twins were in NNU. I was gobsmacked, what mother would leave her fragile babies alone? A month later I found myself in a Thai restaurant, twins safely tucked up in their hospital cots and me tucking into a Thai green chicken curry (mild of course).

I was told very early in pregnancy that there was a high likelihood we'd have to spend some time in the neonatal care unit, later during the pregnancy checking into NNU became a certainty.

Jess and Isla were born at 35 weeks weighing 1,5kg (3lbs 5oz) and 2,45kg (5lbs 8oz) and we stayed in neonatal care for nearly three weeks. Even though there was never a time when I had to rationally fear for their lives or their development these three weeks were an extreme, somewhat scary and at the same time very precious experience. When I first saw Isla I was totally overwhelmed by feelings of happiness and fear. She was so tiny. How did I end up having such a tiny baby? I often find myself remembering those days when she was fragile and too weak to breastfeed. Her eyes were black, her skin was loose and her mouth was too small to even latch on.

Two days after birth, the hospital closed the neonatal unit due to a Norovirus outbreak. It was somehow good that visitors weren't allowed in, as I could put all my time and effort into establishing breastfeeding and changing as many nappies by myself as possible.

I met so many lovely people whilst in hospital. I am still in touch with some of the mums I met there and it's so lovely to keep track of how well their babies are doing, especially those who were born very early. I think we all became quite close as we kind of needed one another. If only I had a photograph of us lot creeping down the corridor to the canteen, there were five of us but only Tash and I have had twins. When we turned up, the canteen ladies greeted us with "oh the hungry twin mums are here" and gave us double portions. And it didn't stop there, we actually went back after dinner just to eat any left over food the dinner ladies had wrapped up and left in the fridge for us to eat. There was a snack machine located next to the fridge and I am not joking when I say that Tash and I had at least four chocolate bars every day on top of the double meals. When the machine had run out of our favourite energy boosters there was another one just outside the hospital reception and the receptionists already knew where we were heading when we came down to exit the hospital for just one minute half way through the night. We ate so much! And we cried so much. But really, there is no better place to cry than the hospital, may it be the neonatal care ward, labour ward or antenatal ward. The nurses, midwives, dinner ladies and cleaners were all so understanding. They see it every day and many of them are mums themselves. If you feel like crying, do it here!

I guess it was a good thing that I knew that at least one of my girls would have to spend time in neonatal care as it gave me the chance to prepare myself. I took part in a hospital visit especially designed for twin parents whilst I was still pregnant and we were given a lot of information about the neonatal unit, incubators, tube feeding, expressing, natural birth and c-sections etc. I did read up on breastfeeding premature babies and how to establish a good supply of milk without actually having a baby to feed. I felt fairly well prepared, but probably only because I knew I had to be. But many expectant twin mums aren't aware of the likelihood of their babies arriving early and a possible stay in neonatal care.

I have spoken to twin mums who were sailing through their pregnancy and all of a sudden, for no apparent reason, the little monkeys decided to make an early appearance. Totally unprepared, shocked and very overwhelmed by the sudden end of the pregnancy they found themselves sat next to two incubators now home to their babies, surrounded by a variety of bleeping machines that constantly trigger alarms which most of the time can be ignored but still get your heart rate up in an instant.

I also met mums who had their babies at full term and yet ended up in neonatal care because of other problems with the babies or problems that occurred during birth. It's a good idea to prepare

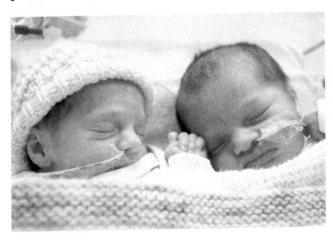

Isla and Jess
a few days old.

yourself for the possibility that you might spend some time in neonatal care.

Had I known then what I know now, I would have read or at least printed the really helpful guides I had found on the Tamba website and on the BLISS website bliss.org.uk. I had downloaded some of them but I didn't bother printing and reading them until several months later. All this info would have been very helpful if only I had read it before the arrival of my tiny premature babies.

When in neonatal care, especially with premature babies, you are confronted with a cocktail of emotions; you might feel lost, helpless, frustrated, cheated, scared, worried and maybe even guilty. All these feelings are normal and you are not alone if you experience them.

KANGAROO CARE – SO MUCH MORE THAN A FUNKY NAME

Kangaroo care is a technique initially developed in areas where incubators were limited, not available or unreliable. Named after the similarity to how a kangaroo mother cares for her baby, this technique is applied to newborn babies, especially premature babies, where the baby is held in skin to skin contact for as long as medically possible.

The idea of the skin to skin contact is to restore the closeness of the womb and has been found to reduce infections and other illnesses but most importantly it significantly reduced mortality rates in less developed areas of our world. It doesn't matter who cuddles, mother or father, it's all about keeping your babies warm, for them to hear your heart beat, smell you, hear you and feel save with you. It's also a really wonderful, peaceful way of bonding with your tiny babies. It promotes breastfeeding and in some cases it feels like it's the only thing you can do – where really it is one of the most beneficial things you can do to help your premature baby.

When reading up on Kangaroo Care I came across something totally amazing: Thermal Synchrony! Now this is something only mums can do: when a baby is placed skin to skin on its mums chest, the temperature of the mother's breasts changes so that her baby can better maintain its own temperature. If the baby is too cold the mother's body temperature will warm up by up to two degrees Celsius within just two minutes. If the baby is too hot, the mother's body temperature will decrease to cool her baby. This is also proven to work when having a lovely double kangaroo cuddle with twins.

*There are many things I remember from our NNU stay.
I remember the first time we held our babies together,
still attached to monitors. I remember the first time I
gave them a kangaroo care cuddle at the same time. I
remember weighing the used nappies. I remember being
so pleased when they put on an oz. I remember that Ethan
at his smallest looked like a little old man and that Sophia
had the biggest eyes I'd ever seen. I could go on forever.
Zoe, mum to Ellis, Sophia and Ethan.*

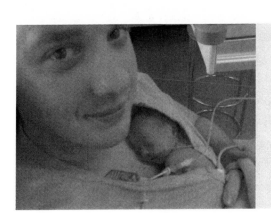

*Tiny Sophia having
a skin to skin cuddle
with daddy Martyn.*

BONDING WITH YOUR BABIES

Early bonding is a lovely idea, the idea that you see your babies and you are overwhelmed with love and closeness is wonderful but reality is not (always) like that.

I remember those awkward moments sat in a wheelchair in front of an incubator looking at that tiny person living in that box, connected to all sorts of pipes and tubes, surrounded by blinking lights and alarms going off... and I waited for that wave of love and closeness to sweep over me but it was just not coming. Just a wave of pain coming from that humongous scar across my tummy and from the after pains caused by my double sized womb shrinking back into near original size (sorry, expectant mums, this probably won't happen to you).

I think early bonding is a bit of a myth, maybe a bit like 'love at first sight'. I am not saying it doesn't exist, all I am saying is that the importance is overrated and you shouldn't beat yourself up for not feeling instant love and closeness. You could fall in love and spend the rest of your life with someone you have already known for years or you could meet someone at a Japanese train station and know he's the one. Same applies for babies. If bonding had to happen straight away, how could anyone ever adopt a toddler or a child?

Feeling a little numb and shocked after the birth and therefore delayed bonding are totally normal, especially if one or both of your babies are in intensive / neonatal care. Things are just different then. It's a strange feeling that the doctors and nurses seem to know your babies much better than you do. You walk in and they tell you: "Oh good morning, Jess has just been for a brain scan and everything looks fine." Or: "Isla has been a really good girl and kept the whole feed down." Or you walk over to the incubator, home to your child for the last week, and suddenly your little bold baby girl has turned into a slightly bigger baby boy with a great deal of brown hair and a blue teddy bear by his feet. A second later I was told that my baby had been moved from special care into high dependency care. Phew!

These moments aren't really helping the whole bonding experience but they are part of life in neonatal care. And there's nothing wrong with them, it's comforting that the nurses know more than you do, it's fine for you to take a nap when your babies are being fed or checked up on, you don't need to be there for everything, for every feed (unless you are ready to establish breastfeeding), for every nappy. If you feel like you can and if you want to then that's great but if you feel like you need a rest then do so. You have a fair number of nappies to change and feeds to give in the months and years ahead, get some rest now, look after yourself, don't overdo it. Your babies are in very special care, with the best qualified babysitters you'll ever get! When we finally left hospital I wished I could just stuff Nurse Tracy in my hospital bag, take her home and keep her forever.

Don't hold your bonding expectations too high. Talk to your babies. Tell people around you how you feel, tell them about your babies, talk to other twin mums and just wait and see. One step at a time.

"I spent such a long time in hospital (five different ones in the South West), six and a half weeks before giving birth and then the boys spent the same length of time in NNU. I only really started to bond with the boys when I took them home and I first found myself alone with them."
Julie, mum to Holly, Harrison and Daniel

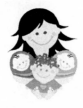

Older Siblings

Jacob had just turned three when I checked into NNU and I missed him so much. The hospital wasn't that far away and Jacob and daddy tried to come and visit every day. Unfortunately the ward closure also affected siblings and they weren't allowed to visit either. Jacob couldn't even see his two little sisters to help him understand why his Mummy wasn't at home to put him to bed, give him breakfast or watch "Lunar Jim" with him. All this talk about the two sisters in mummy's tummy and then the tummy is gone and no babies to be seen. It must have been very hard to understand for a three year old.

Whilst the girls were still tube fed with my expressed milk, I did take the opportunity to escape for a few hours to go home and just spent a few hours snuggled up on the couch with my little boy. I cried my eyes out when heading back to the hospital and at the same time couldn't wait to get there as a totally irrational worry about my babies had crept up on me whilst I had been away. Later when I was feeding

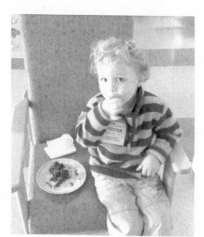

Jacob brought some cake for the nurses and doctors on the neonatal ward; and himself of course.

the babies every three hours I didn't have any chance to visit Jacob at home but one afternoon the nurse noticed how much I missed my little boy and offered to give the girls a full tube feed and therefore I was able to leave the hospital for five hours – Rich, Jacob and I went to an adventure park and on a train ride. It was just wonderful and I felt so revitalised and so happy when I got back to the hospital.

Jacob was really impressed that his newborn baby sisters had managed to get him a present despite being in hospital and living in plastic boxes and all. He still remembers it two years later.

It was a wonderful moment, when he first held his tiny little baby sisters; he was so gentle with them. All through the pregnancy I had told him to be very careful with Jess's and Isla's bump-home, he was allowed to very carefully place his ear on my bump and try to listen to them and sometimes he would very gently feel them move around.

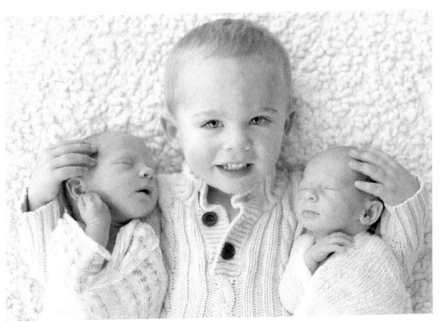

Big brother Oliver very carefully holding his newborn twin sisters Vivian and Sydney © Jamie Ibey of I See Beauty Photography

DEALING WITH A TRAUMATIC PREGNANCY OR BIRTH

In most cases it doesn't matter how the pregnancy and birth went, as the outcome, two babies, simply makes up for any pain you went through to get there. I had a stressful pregnancy and life in neonatal care was an intense experience, but it was far from traumatic. Even those with much more stressful experiences than mine were much too busy, happy and relieved as to actually stop and comprehend what had happened. But sometimes these experiences sit too deep and can't just be ignored as they may lead to a post traumatic stress disorder.

A good starting point for anyone thinking they might be affected in the UK is the Birth Trauma Association. www. birthtraumaassociation.org.uk

Jodi Kluchar runs a group in the US. www.angelfire.com/moon2/jkluchar1995/

Penny Christianson runs Birth Trauma Canada. http://birthtraumacanada.org.

HELD in Australia run a popular Facebook page. www.facebook.com/BirthTraumaAustralia

BIRTH STORIES

MAX and OSCAR, born at 27 weeks gestation, weighing 980g (2lbs 2oz) and 960g (2lbs 1oz), written by mum Georgina

Frank and I found out I was expecting identical twins at week seven after some spotting made us go to the early pregnancy unit. We were shocked and bemused. My grandfather was a non-identical twin so it was always a running joke that one of the grandkids would have twins. We were then under the watchful eye of Professor Nicolaides and his team because of the risk of Twin to Twin Transfusion Syndrome (TTTS) in identical twins. We had scans every two weeks from then on. At 14 weeks I had a bleed and throughout our pregnancy there were worries about twin one (Oscar) because of excess fluid in the ventricles of his brain. We were told at every scan that there was a chance he may be severely brain damaged.

At week 27+1 we were at home with my dad putting together cots when I noticed I was having regular cramps. I didn't really think anything was wrong but phoned the midwives at 5.30pm and was told to come in to see what was going on. I told my dad that we'd see him in a few hours and to put our food delivery away if we weren't home when it came at 8pm.

We got to the hospital and I was told I was having contractions and was taken to the labour ward where things happened very quickly. At 10pm I was examined and I was 7cm dilated, scrubs were thrown at Frank and we were taken down for an emergency c-section.

The boys were born at 10.21pm and 10.24pm. There were two teams from the neonatal unit ready for the boys and they took them away. I caught a brief glimpse of them. Frank saw them an hour later in the unit.

Oscar was moved to St Thomas for the first few days because

they didn't have the room in the unit.

My best friends and family saw him before I did!

I remember seeing Max for the first time and feeling scared and numb. He didn't look like a baby, he was scrawny and bruised. He had so many wires and tubes surrounding him. It was terrifying. I had a very strong maternal sense though at that moment. I've never been a broody person, never cooed over babies but this little man had me straight away and he was so fragile.

I felt so helpless when the boys were in the incubators. Luckily I produced plenty of milk over the next few days and was determined to make it work for them. It was the only thing I could do! I had my first cuddle with Max after a week and Oscar a few days later. It was amazing and scary at the same time. They had so many wires I was terrified I'd pull something out so I sat very still. We had a relatively easy ride considering how early the boys were born. They were early but had no additional problems when born. Oscar was monitored regarding his ventricles; they never got bigger and haven't been a problem since.

The boys did well and after being in hospital for eight weeks there was talk of Max coming home, he was off the oxygen. He then caught an infection and was taken back to intensive care for three days before making a full recovery and coming home two weeks

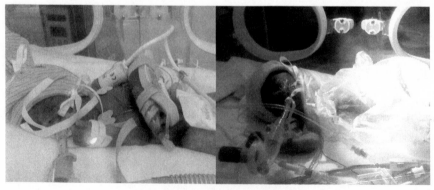

Tiny babies, Max and Oscar.

later. Oscar also caught the infection and actually went blue and stopped breathing in my arms, something I was reminded about by my Frank when thinking of what to write for this book. Obviously I'd blanked that from my memory. He was whisked off and was back in intensive care for three days as well, always a day behind Max in terms of recovery. They both came home ten weeks later. We placed them in their car seats on our dining table and both stood there not knowing what to do next!

The boys have developed really well. They came home weighing 5lbs and have never really put a lot of weight on. They were and are thin but have very healthy appetites. The first year was unbelievably tiring and quite stressful (we moved when they were eight months old to be close to our families). I was told by health visitors that they were too small and thin, and then told by the doctors they were fine. I didn't know what to think as a new mum and doubted my own instincts. In the end I told our paediatrician that I would see him only and that I was sick and tired of being told my boys weren't doing well when I felt, as a mum, that they were fine.

They are now two and a half and have just been signed off by the paediatrician. They are two very cheeky, loving and active boys. I love the age they are at the moment and Oscar, despite all the early concerns about his brain is a very bright and chatty young man. They both amaze me and make me smile from ear to ear every day!

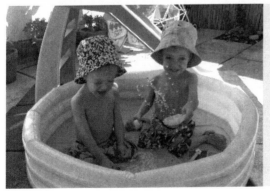

Max and Oscar two years old.

SOPHIA and ETHAN, born at 30 weeks gestation, weighing 1500g (3lbs 5oz) and 1590g (3lbs 8 oz), written by mum Zoe

We found out that we were expecting twins pretty early on due to some early bleeding, it was this bleeding that made me feel a little wary and led to me keeping it to myself as long as possible. At 22 weeks I told our eldest son, Ellis. I didn't really have a lot of choice after this comment when he saw me in the shower, "mummy your tummy is getting so big, have you got a baby in there?"

We were monitored quite closely and had regular scans. On the whole this was a good thing until during one scan they noticed an "ecogenic bowel". The consultant did not seem overly concerned and said that he would review at the next scan. After a couple of emotional weeks waiting for the next scan, thankfully everything was fine. Looking back I unfortunately felt quite nervous throughout the whole pregnancy and regret that I never just took the time to enjoy it.

After an internal scan of my cervix I was being told that my cervix was very short in length, shorter than they would like. Another scan was planned for two weeks to compare. I did show no real change. However the next one, two weeks later again showed another dramatic reduction which led to the consultant suggesting some rest and I was therefore signed off from work until another scan two weeks later.

This scan was on Christmas eve. My cervix was only showing as 1 mm, I was only 26 weeks pregnant, my consultant felt that I could go into labour at any time and decided for me to be admitted. Worried is probably an understatement, and to be honest not only for me but for Ellis too. Father Christmas was due in the morning and at just 5 years old I didn't want this to be ruined for him. Luckily as we lived so close to the hospital it was agreed that I could go home, make the evening and morning as special as possible and return to the hospital once all presents had been opened. Just before we left I had to have some steroids that would improve the babies' lung development in order to give them the best possible chance of survival. That certainly made it hit home that 26 weeks was definitely too early. The following morning, I went back to the hospital and had my second steroid injection. This certainly wasn't how I wanted to spend my Christmas day.

Amazingly we reached 28 weeks and I came home on the 7th Jan but unfortunately only for a week as I started to bleed quite heavily and rushed back into hospital. Following numerous checks, monitors and quite a lot of waiting I was told that I was not in labour, the babies were not distressed and that they ultimately wanted them to stay inside me for as long as possible. I went home once the bleeding had stopped on the 24th Jan, however this time only for a total of seven hours. The bleeding started again and I rushed back to the hospital where my consultant told me that this time I would not be going anywhere - I didn't argue.

Finally on the 26th Jan I think my body just decided enough was enough, the bleeding started again and this time very heavy.

The next ten minutes involved a number of checks, questions and monitoring. I was asked how I would like to deliver my twins and by this time, feeling very helpless, in a lot of discomfort I said that although

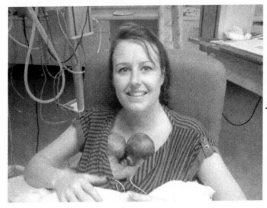

Zoe giving Sophia and Ethan kangaroo cuddles.

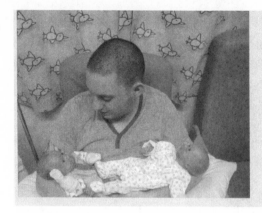

Daddy Martyn holding his tiny babies Sophia and Ethan.

originally I wanted a natural birth I just wanted them to do whatever they needed to make this as safe as possible for me and my babies. This was an emergency c-section, however during this conversation I went from not being in labour, to being in labour and 5 cm dilated. It was suddenly all hands on deck. The next thing I know is my contractions were very constant, I was in theatre and surrounded by people. I was told when each of my babies was lifted out and I heard their little cries which was an amazing feeling.

I was able to have a very quick glimpse of my baby girl before she was rushed to intensive care. Ethan needed a little oxygen straight

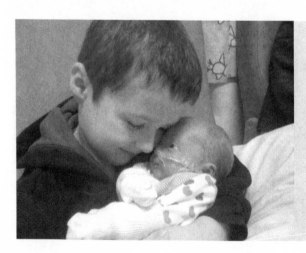

Big brother Ellis carefully cuddling his tiny baby sister Sophia.

away so I had to wait a little longer to see his gorgeous little face.

My first proper look at my babies was a photo that Martyn took on his phone; due to the loss of blood I had to spend some time recuperating.

Obviously it's not how you want your first glance of your babies to be and I don't really know what I was expecting but, they were my babies and they were gorgeous.

So for the next four and a half weeks we spent our time going back and forwards from the hospital to home. We were very lucky, our journey on the NNU went very smoothly, I was continually amazed.

On the 28th Feb Ethan weighing just 4lb 13 and Sophia 4lb 14, my gorgeous twins came home.

Two years on we have two bouncing, cheeky, mischievous little toddlers. Sophia may have had reflux and Ethan may have to wear glasses but I am not convinced that this is anything to do with their prematurity. What I am convinced of however is that my rollercoaster journey has ended with an amazing two additions to our family.

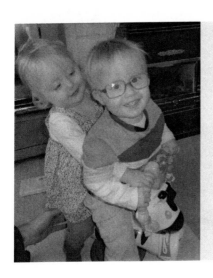

Toddling Sophia and Ethan loving life.

HARRISON and DANIEL, born at 30 weeks gestation, weighing 1615g (3lb 9oz) and 1815g (4lbs)

Harrison and Daniel were born at 30 weeks gestation after Julie's waters went at 23 weeks and four days on twin two - Daniel.

At birth Harrison (twin one) was 3lb 9oz and Daniel (twin two) was 4lbs and they remained in NNU for six and a half weeks. Mum Julie stayed with them for about ten days after they were born and then went to "room in" with them for about a week before they came home.

Harrison and Daniel have an older sister called Holly who had to be without her mummy for quite sometime before and after the birth of her baby brothers. It was quite a challenge organising childcare and they roped in all their family and friends.

Two years later and Holly still recalls her mum's absence, whenever they pass their local Indian restaurant she exclaims: "This is where daddy took me in my pyjamas when you were in hospital". Once the boys were born, Holly came to visit her baby brothers in neonatal care wearing her nurse dress up, which must have been incredibly cute and I bet all the NNU nurses loved her. Despite their early start to life the boys are doing great and have just started school.

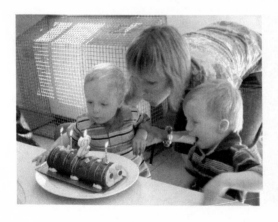

Daniel and Harrison celebrating their second birthday with mum Julie at Twinsclub.

STAN and ELSIE, born at 38 weeks gestation, weighing 2860g (6lbs 5oz) and 2980g (6lbs 9oz)

We found out we were having twins at the 12 week scan, my bump was already massive and friends had been joking that I might be expecting twins. And then we got the confirmation, twins! I went back home and cried; George went back to work but was sent home soon after as he was in too much of a state. Our daughter Lily was going to be 21 months when they were due and we were living in a tiny cottage. But shock soon turned into excitement.

I read a few books about twin births and decided that I really didn't want a c-section. Lily's birth had been natural and I didn't like the prospect of being stuck with a 21 months old and twin babies whilst recovering from a c-section. I spoke to the consultant and he agreed that given that we were all well at the time I could deliver them naturally. The pregnancy was smooth without any complications. My bump was huge but I pretty much sailed through it. Both babies were always in a head down position, as if they too were also set on a natural delivery.

At 38 weeks I had a sweep, the midwives told me that I was actually three cm dilated, but nothing happened and after a while they sent me home. In the evening I started to have side pains on my bump, they didn't feel like contractions at all, I phoned the hospital and was told to come in. The monitors showed that I was having contractions, but I wasn't feeling anything. I did the things you do when you're in labour, sat on the ball for a while, waited for something to happen but after a while the alleged contractions stopped. An anaesthetist came in to prep me, I told him that I was planning to give birth without an epidural, a short while later and I was screaming for him to come back and give me an epidural, which he did. I was in full blown labour and forever fiddling with the leads of the monitors that kept falling off when I moved around. It took ages, at one point George asked the midwife "At what point are we considering a c-section?" and she replied: "Oh we are nowhere near that point." Stan was eventually born first at 23:30pm on the 5th of June. His sister Elsie took her time. She was back to back now and after a little break and then a lot of pulling Elsie was born at 0:30am on the 6th of June.

I breastfed them straight away and they were both very well. They didn't have to go into the neonatal unit and stayed in the room with me. Two days later we went home. My in-laws offered to put us up whilst we were looking for a bigger house and we lived with them for a year and they were brilliant, especially with Lily. I always knew she was well looked after and I tried to sleep as much as possible. Stan and Elsie were really good babies, they slept well, they fed well and once I had cracked tandem feeding life was getting much easier. Maybe they were feeding so well because there was an element of competition. They used to smile at one another on the feeding pillow and hold hands, it was so lovely. They make each other laugh so much and they love each other dearly. They always slept together and they slept so well. When we eventually got them their own beds, they pushed them together to make one big bed. I don't really remember much of the first year or two, it was hard and you don't really get the time to think about it. You're in a bubble and you just have to get on with it. It's hilarious they are twins but don't share a birthday.

Stan and Elsie
snuggled up for a
daytime nap.

MY DIARY
ISLA'S AND JESS'S BIRTH
AND OUR STAY IN
NEONATAL CARE

Tuesday, 16th March. – The Day X

Rich's mum arrives at 7 am at our house and I kiss my little boy goodbye. Rich and I head off to hospital to have two babies. It feels surreal. My body is knackered, my feet are so swollen that I had to cut the sides of my trainers in order to make them fit, I can no longer move my feet due to all the water retention, I can only guess where my kneecaps might be residing as it's all swollen around them too. My hands (also huge!) have been numb for weeks, my bump measures 113cm, I weigh 92.7 kg and I can barely get onto my feet. I am so ready to end this pregnancy in a royal caesarean way this morning.

We arrive at the hospital on time which is a good start and are taken to a room on the labour ward for preparations, a lovely midwife called Jess is with us; she will later tell everyone that we named one of the girls after her, which isn't true but still a lovely story. I had been visiting the hospital every single day last week, for my steroid injections, for another scan, because I couldn't feel Isla move and one afternoon because I actually had regular contractions which luckily stopped.

We put our scrubs on, midwife Jess helps me squeeze my elephant legs into stockings, and I go to the toilet a million times. Quick cardiotocography (CTG) to check the girls are ok, then the surgeons arrive to talk us through the c-section. Everyone is cheerful and alert and I think to myself that it's always a good sign if a surgeon doesn't look tired. The two anaesthetists come in and tell us all about the combined epidural - spinal block they will be using. As my girls share the placenta the c-section may take longer than expected and the epidural will allow them to top up the anaesthetics if needed.

Everyone knows exactly what they are doing; we take a few fun photos and then it's show time. We walk to the theatre and bump into our consultant. "What are you doing here?" he jokes. We enter the theatre and there are so many people here, Rich later counts 20 in total but further medical students and midwives appear to be popping in now and then. Everyone's in a good mood, we say our "hellos" and I am asked to sit down on the table. The anaesthetist checks my back and the lovely two midwives are still beside us. The anaesthetist is inserting a drip into my hand and I avoid seeing it and look over to the nurses who are just positioning two cots for my girls – wow, I will actually be having two babies in a moment! It's just after 9am now, I am asked to curl my back but it's really difficult with this big bump plus one of the babies appears to be engaged. The anaesthetist makes some drawings on my back, applies a sticky sheet to my back, administers local anaesthetics with three little injections and then starts to place the spinal. It's quite intense and I sent Rich away as I think I need to do this on my own. Our chosen music starts playing, Kathryn Jenkins.

The anaesthetist starts but it's not going very well, a massive pain shoots down my right side, it's so painful – I start shaking all over and regret that I sent Rich away. I ask for someone to come over and hold my arm, and someone does. The anaesthetist tries again but no success. His senior colleague takes over, finds a different vertebrate and within minutes the spinal and epidural are in place and the pain gone. The junior anaesthetist must have felt so awful and I felt really sorry for him too. I guess he was just nervous too. He makes up for it in every possible way as he stays with us throughout the birth, he sits next to my head and is our running commentary for everything that's happening or about to happen. They insert a catheter and we are ready to go. I am lying down on the table now but in a weird way, tilted to the left, surely I will fall off this table any minute but magically I don't. The screen is being put up and Rich sits down to the right of my head. He nearly fainted during the spinal-procedure and had been taken to a small room next door, but he was back on track now. There is a big monitor next to him and he has to move forwards a bit, unwillingly allowing him to look past the screen and see everything.

I take deep breaths and go into my own little zone. The surgeon paints my bump and they get all the instruments ready. My voice is gone now. I let it all happen, I feel a bit funny when they do the cut, keep on breathing, all is good. Not long and the anaesthetist tells Rich that it's time to get the camera ready. Here comes our first baby girl, and what a grand entrance she makes, she screams at the top of her lungs - Jess is born! I can feel my bump go down, a really funny feeling as all the pressure has disappeared now. Rich takes the most amazing picture which I am sharing with you here.

The surgeons cut the cord, and carefully place the end still attached to my placenta onto my tummy. Jess's cord is clamped, she

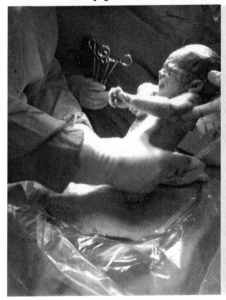

The moment
Jess is born
into this world.

is placed in a cot and off she goes to the resuscitation station.

Now it's Isla's turn, the small twin, the one I am so worried about. She must have figured out by now that something was going on. I actually know exactly what happens now as my amazing husband filmed it with my phone! The surgeons find Isla's bottom and gently pull it out, they take her feet and stretch her, they find her head and then pull her out, upside down stretching her little body and two minutes after her big sister, Isla is born! They place her on my now amazingly flat and empty tummy, her eyes are wide open and she is waving her arms around. She doesn't cry and I don't know if she is okay, Rich tells me she is fine, I am so relieved and happy. This part is done, they're out! They're born and they are alert and both seem to be doing well. I tell Rich to go and see them. We discussed this in advance. I don't expect to cuddle them or see much of them for the first few hours. Rich will follow them to the Neonatal Unit (NNU) and will find me in the recovery room later.

The surgeons are chatting about some new band and joking about finding a third baby but I can't speak, my throat is so dry. The anaesthetist gives me a tiny little plastic tube with sterilised water and it's the best drink I have ever had in my life. My tummy is being

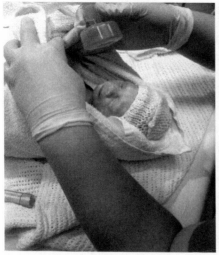

*Isla at the resuscitation
table receiving
a little oxygen.*

stitched up and the girls are now ready to be taken to NNU, I get to take a quick look at them but ask the nurses to just take them to NNU please, I will have my whole life with them. I just want them to be looked after now. The surgeons finish and I am being taken to the recovery room. Lots of people offer congratulations and it still feels very surreal. I sleep a little while and then Rich is back with pictures and the video. Amazing. He is my hero. The midwives come to help express colostrum. They show me how to hand express and between the three of us we express a total of 62ml – I am a legend for a day as this is a huge amount.

I phone my parents and post a little message on the internet at 11:30am. I sleep a bit more and at 2pm one of the nurses pushes my bed over to NNU where I meet my parents, and my twins! Jess is in intensive care, in an incubator, wearing nothing but a nappy and she is on Continuous Positive Airway Pressure (CPAP). This is applied via a small mask over her nose and helps the air sacs in her lungs to stay open. Isla is in high dependency care next door. She's in an incubator too, just in a nappy and breathing without assistance. Both have drips in their tiny hands and lots of little monitoring leads stuck to their chest and feet.

She is tiny and I start to cry. Never before in my life have I seen

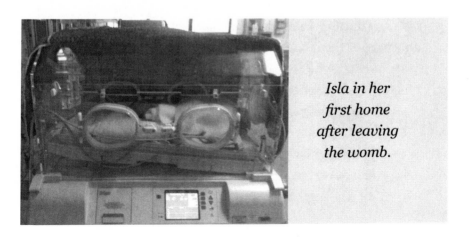

Isla in her first home after leaving the womb.

such a tiny person. She weighs only 1.5kg (3lbs 5) and is 41cm tall. Her eyes are black and wide open and she is looking at me. She is beautiful. I can't really see much of Jess as she is on the CPAP. She weighs 2.45 kg (5lbs 8) and is around 48cm.

It's all very overwhelming. Jacob, Rich and Granny come in to see them. I am being taken back to my room, Rich brings my bags and I sleep a bit. I make another visit later in the afternoon. I express some more colostrum and thanks to a shot glass of diamorphine sleep all through the night - unfortunately, as I was supposed to express every three hours.

Wednesday 17th March

On my first morning of being a twin mum I have to wait for the drip and catheter to be removed, two lovely nurses come and help me out of bed and I have a shower, feels great! I can hardly move, the scar is huge and my bump is still massive but the shower feels wonderful. My feet and legs have swollen even more, this body looks very funny, maybe I should avoid the mirror in the bathroom :) I get in the wheelchair and one of the nurses takes me over to NNU to see my babies. Jess is no longer on CPAP and I stroke her through the holes in the incubator. I also get to have a proper cuddle with her. She is beautiful too and she enjoys the cuddle very much.

Rich and Jacob join us and Rich has a cuddle with Isla. The boys brought cake for the labour ward staff, NNU and the maternity ward – they are very popular. It's lovely to see them. I miss my little Jacob very much already. I ask to be wheeled over to see the girls a few more times and back in the room I try to express but with little success. I panic a little bit as I am determined to breastfeed my babies and decide to express regularly through the night, but I am so exhausted and in so much pain that I end up taking diamorphine and sleeping all through the night again.

Thursday 18th March

I am a failure, and a mess. I should have expressed last night but I didn't; now I get near to nothing when I express. 0.5ml – that's all. The girls are now formula fed. I have to relax and get a grip on expressing. I am worried about little Isla, she is so tiny, she needs my milk, not formula. Jess is out of the incubator and now in a hot cot. Her drip has been removed and she is now in high dependency care, right next to her sister. They are increasing both their feeds which is great. I express every three hours and in the evening I express 1ml – devastated! A new girl moves into my room and she is my saviour. Caz has had baby number three, a baby girl born prematurely and Caz has to express breast milk too – but Caz has a major advantage, she has done it twice before as all her babies had arrived early. And she knows exactly what to do and I just tag on to her and do what she does, express when she does. I try expressing by hand again but quickly resort back to the electrical pump. Still not a lot but I just keep going and in the middle of night proudly take my 2ml of gold dust across to NNU. It must be so comical watching these totally knackered new mums making their way to the neonatal ward, in the middle of the night looking a right mess, handing over their precious 2ml of colostrum and all the nurses smile at them and praise them "that's great, you've done reeeeally well." It's hilarious – if only it wasn't so serious.

I have been an emotional wreck all day. I crept along the corridors, crying my eyes out. Got a cuddle from the dinner lady, the NNU nurse and a random lady working on the maternity ward. She went on to tell me that she was born prematurely in the fifties, weighing only 3 lbs (1.36kg). She claims she has never had any problems and that she was actually a very smart and strong woman. She even ran the London marathon. How caring of her, to share this with me. Everyone's lovely and I can barely say a sentence without bursting into tears. The scar hurts and I need to remember to take my painkillers in a timely manner. Last night, when I slept all through the night, the nurse looking after the girls made a diary entry around 8pm that Jess was wanting a breastfeed and that mum (Me!) was nowhere to be found. Trust me, there's no way I could possibly feel any guiltier than I did after reading that comment. Then of course, I didn't manage to turn up the entire night thanks to the power of diamorphine – but hey that was last night, now there's Caz in my room and I'll just do what she does. Bring on the sleepless nights.

Friday, 19th March

The only way is up! I expressed at midnight, 3am and 6am, not much but we're getting there. Jess had a good go at breastfeeding this morning. I have been up since 3am with the girls, nappy changing, feeding, expressing... a taste of what's to come? I hope not. Slept a little bit from 6am to 8:45am. The doctor came to see me; I am well enough now to be discharged. I can stay on the ward though and get myself on the waiting list for a parent's room in NNU. That's great news. I will definitely stay, I am really getting somewhere with breastfeeding Jess now and live too far away to just return for feeds. We have a permanent parking ticket now which is great.

Isla is off the drip by 11am, the consultant looks at her and says to the nurse: "Get rid of it right now, she doesn't need it anymore!" Her poor little hand is all blue and bruised.

Rich and Jacob are picking me up at 4pm. We were planning to go to a Japanese restaurant but end up going home instead which is lovely. So many cards to congratulate us, I don't even know some of the people who made the effort to send a card. I hand express a bit at home, just to stick to my routine. I have a wonderful cuddle with my little Jacob on our couch watching some kids television. At 7pm we get in the car and the boys take me back to hospital. I start crying in the car, I miss my little boy so much. I hope we'll all be home soon and have a big family cuddle.

Saturday 20th March

Last night's expressing went very well, I got myself a door opening pass for the night and no longer have to wait for randomly passing nurses to let me in or out of the ward. Jess had her first proper breastfeed at 1am in the night, I feel so proud! I am getting used to hospital life, got to know quite a few other mums. I express next to the babies now which works much better. I have my own steriliser in the "milk kitchen", I get my shields and pipes and some bottles from the milk kitchen first, then grab one of the wheelie tables with a double breast pump on and roll it over to the room where my girls are. Jess is in a normal cot and I just take her out when I express and breastfeed her on one side whilst expressing from the other. At night I use the double pump function and let her sleep and grow, she will have my milk straight after expressing it via their feeding tubes, it's at the perfect temperature for them.

I am expressing enough to feed both girls most of the time. The nurse tonight is a mum of twins and she has tons of good advice for me, she changes their feeding times so they are in sync which makes life much easier. Jacob is staying at his cousins' tonight, I haven't seen him all day but I will see him tomorrow, I hope he is okay. Gosh, do I miss my little man. Rich is out tonight with some friends, feels strange how different our lives have become, I am up every three hours to feed and express and only getting 90 minute chunks of sleep whilst he is living the life.

Sunday, 21st March

From 7am the girls are no longer in high dependency but low dependency care. Isla has moved out of her incubator and is now in a warm cot equipped with a warm water mattress and we have moved two rooms down the corridor, two rooms closer to the exit. I am expressing and feeding Jess at the same time. Nurse I. (let's keep her anonymous) is in charge of the girls today and she is no where to be seen. I can't find her anywhere for the 12am feed, by 12:30 I give up searching for her and ask one of the other nurses to give my girls their tube feed. When she eventually turns up she is very apologetic but I decide to stay around all day as I really don't trust her. This morning she gave Jess formula through the feeding tube (Jess still gets a top up after breastfeeding) literally a minute before I finished expressing. She just pours the formula into the syringe whilst I sit right next to her. I could have just interrupted and handed over my warm breast milk, it would have taken seconds to do that and after all that is the reason I am expressing my milk. If I wanted them to have formula I wouldn't be sat here with my milking machine. I was so upset. I had made it quite clear that I just wanted to use breast milk now and I was expressing more than enough now anyway. I explain my frustration and she seems to get it. After the 4pm feed Rich picks me up and we head home for a Sunday roast, Jacob gives me the best cuddle ever when he sees me and eats his dinner sitting on my lap. I love him so much.

I get a lift back to the hospital, tonight's nurse is Tracey, she is a nursing nurse and finally someone who is willing to talk facts. She thinks Isla will be in NNU for another three weeks as she needs all her energy to put on weight. Breastfeeding her just results in her using too much energy to feed, energy she needs to just grow right now. Tracey wants to see how Jess is feeding and she is very pleased with it and thinks Jess could be heading home in a week's time. We discuss the criteria for going home and work out a feeding and expressing schedule. At night I feed Jess and express at the same time, every four hours. She then gets a top up via tube with milk from the same breast in order for her to get the hind milk. We then put her back to bed. If she stirs, Tracey settles her and sends me straight back to bed. No fussing with Isla, we just let her sleep. And I get, surprisingly, a lot of sleep. Jess is so funny when she is hungry, she gets so grumpy and loud, she is such a feisty little girl. She needs to gain weight in order for her tube top ups to be reduced and she is being weighed tomorrow.

Monday, 22nd March

Jess hasn't gained weight but not to worry. Nurse Ellen is looking after the girls today and I tell her all about Jacob and she comes up with a cunning plan how he can get a glimpse of the girls despite the closure of the ward due to a Norovirus outbreak on another ward. It turns out to be major success. In the afternoon I go out with Jacob and Rich to feed swans and ducks. Tracey is doing the night shift and again I manage to get a lot of sleep. We discuss more details of the "taking Jess home plan". Jess needs to:

- have gained weight on Wednesday in order for tube top ups to be reduced

- pass a hearing test and pass a car seat stress test; she'll have to sit in a car seat for one hour whilst her oxygen levels are being monitored

- be exclusively breast fed on Friday, Saturday and Sunday and gain weight

And then the doctor in charge Monday morning might decide that she is free to go. I will come in as often as possible to see Isla who is expected to stay for at least another two weeks. Easter holidays begin next week and therefore there will be no preschool for Jacob. By then I will have been away from him for two weeks so I feel it might be good to come home. At night I sweat so much, I have to actually get changed into dry clothes. But my feet and knees look so much better. I guess this finally marks the end of the nuisance called "water retention".

Tuesday, 23rd March

The night went really well, four hourly feeds are such a luxury! My legs and feet are "back". Feels good. Jess is having a brain scan this morning as she was on CPAP for the first hours of her life – it's a routine procedure. The sonographer applies some jelly onto Jess's fontanelle, also called the soft spot, and scans through the spot. It's like peeping through a keyhole, once the soft spot is closed it becomes no longer possible to look at the brain in such an easy way. Jess sleeps right through her little head massage. All is good. She wakes a little early for her afternoon feed which is a good sign, she is feeding so well with long, strong sucks, she's got it all sussed. She is so sweet and yet so grumpy. Isla has a couple of suckles whilst being tube fed. Every time the housekeeping ladies arrive they gather around Isla's cot and coo over her as they think that Isla looks like a petite little doll in her knitted cardigans.

I go home for a few hours in the evening, cuddle up with my little boy and watch "Lunar Jim". Back at the hospital Tracey is cuddling a hungry Jess, apparently up since 7pm waiting for her 8pm feed – this girl is demanding. I think I need to get used to the fact that I am now a mum of three little children and I have to make them all happy! I feed her and Rich joins later for a cuddle with Jess, whilst Isla is having a suckle during her tube feed. Lots of cuddles later we put the girls to bed, take their beds back to my room on NNU

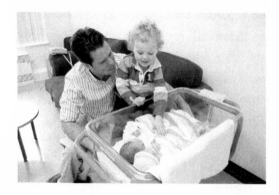

*Jacob visiting
his little baby
sisters Isla and Jess.*

(I am now a lodger and have one of the parent's rooms in the neonatal care unit). We snuggle up and watch "Friends", it's been ages since we've last been alone and I feel like a teenager having my first boyfriend visit my room for the first time. Jess wants a cuddle too and snores away on daddy's chest. At 10pm Rich heads back home, we move the girls back and I go and raid the fridge in the canteen and then go to sleep. During the night I sweat so much that I need to get changed twice and change the bed covers. This is the end of fluid retention and harmless. Slightly disgusting though but hey, my legs are slim, I can see my ankles, my face looks normal again and people have commented on how well I look which feels great.

Wednesday, 24th March

Jess has gained weight! Yes! She is still not back to her birth weight but that doesn't matter, she just needed to gain weight for the top ups to be reduced. That's one box checked on the "get me out of here" list. Today's nurse Louise reduces her top ups drastically. Jess feeds well but I guess those four hourly feeds will be a thing of the past now. She passes her hearing test – another box checked. I am going to miss her 4pm feed as I am going to a park with Jacob and Rich and she will be having her last ever full tube feed. I am so looking forward to seeing my boys. Rich is doing an amazing job, being mummy and daddy at the same time. I get back at 6pm and the girls are fast asleep.

Isla must have overheard all the talk about Jess going home without her and she decides that she can do it too! She latches on and off we go, the little wibbler is feeding like a pro. Amazing. Tonight's night nurse seems very tired which stresses me. She doesn't take Isla's huge breastfeed into consideration and squeezes the whole 51ml top up plus way too much air down her tube and little Isla is being really sick as a result. I hold her whilst she vomits and it's awful. Next feed she barely reduces the tube feed and Isla is sick again. I believe her tummy is too tiny for all that milk but I don't want to stop her on the breast now that she's finally got the hang of it. I am up most of the night, two hungry babies, lots and lots of nappies, lots of pukes but also lots of cuddles with my gorgeous little girls.

Thursday, 25th March

By the morning we have reduced Isla's top ups to 20ml. She is doing so well and she is sleeping for four hours between feeds. I have tried feeding them at the same time but they are still too little, I have to hold their heads in place when I feed them and this is kind of a two-handed job at the moment plus they are not really keen on the rugby hold. Feeding both and changing their nappies takes around 80 minutes, phew. Isla is moved out of the hot cot into an ordinary cot.

I go to the registry office to register their births, how exciting. Jess and Isla swapped birth order during pregnancy, Jess who was twin 2 all along was born first and somehow all the details are muddled up. But the registrar just changes them and I wander back to the hospital with correct names and birth times on my two certificates. Back at the hospital Isla has another brilliant feed and the doctor in charge suggest that I stay another week as there might be a slight chance of both girls going home in a week's time due to Isla's sudden breastfeeding success. I hate the thought of leaving Isla behind anyway so I agree right away. Jess's tube feeds are dropped completely now and she continues to sleep for three to four hours. The freezer is filling up with my expressed milk and we barely use any now. Rich and Jacob come to visit in the afternoon and it's lovely, as always. Later I go for dinner with the other NNU mums and we talk top ups, expressing and baby weights – we're in our own little world. Tonight's nurse is bright awake and very hands on – that's great.

Friday, 26th March

Isla has lost weight. They say that babies initially lose weight when they first start breastfeeding, surely all that puking hasn't helped either. Isla is much more active now and using extra energy. The doctor is concerned and puts her top ups back up. I feed her and then hold her on my shoulder whilst she gets her top up, this time warmed up. Last night the nurse didn't warm it up and Isla appeared to struggle for ages. I am going to put all expressed milk into the freezer now and express for Isla's top ups as and when needed, this way the milk should always be at the perfect temperature. I am here for every top up anyway.

I am officially being discharged today. I still have quite strong after pains, I even pulled the emergency cord whilst in the rest room but apparently it's all normal. I take a nap and nurse Rachel comes to wake me when the girls wake for their feed. Both at the same time! Who to feed first? I need to feed them at the same time! I can't choose between them. I tandem feed them for the first time and Caz walks in and exclaims: "You are amazing!" and that is exactly how I feel! The other NNU mums get dinner for me as I have my hands full. A saying I am sure to be hearing a lot of in the future. Jess passes the car seat test (check). Jacob and Rich come to visit and at night I am up five times to feed my hungry customers. Hard work.

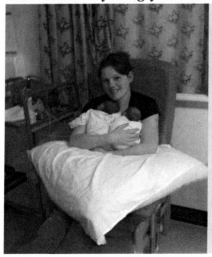

Time for double cuddles.

Saturday, 27th March

Another week in hospital. Isla feeds very well, she latches on and off she goes, she feeds for 15-20 minutes with gentle but very efficient sucks. Day goes well, feeding my babies, chatting to lots of people, I even head into town to buy nappies and a present for Jacob for the evening. Rich and Jacob are in at 6pm but they are both tired and hungry and they head back when it's feeding time for the girls – that makes three hungry children and two knackered parents. I have a busy night and my dreams are so confusing. I dream that nurse Fi comes into my room to tell me that it's time to feed the girls. The dream is so real that I actually wake up, get ready and walk over to find my girls fast asleep and Fi asking me what I am doing here. This happens twice. When Fi really comes to wake me I nearly have a heart attack. I still sweat so much at night, surely all that water retention business must be sorted soon? Tracey does the morning shift, when she comes to wake me at 8:30am I decide it's just a dream and she has to return and wake me a second time. Jess's tube is removed and she has gained 20 grams since yesterday – there is a light at the end of the tunnel!

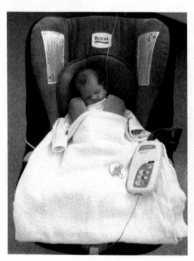

*Jess sleeps right through
her car seat test.*

Sunday, 28th March

Jess gained another 34 grams and that's brilliant but still I am hitting rock bottom today – maybe it's because it's the pain or the sleep deprivation or the fact that it's Rich and my anniversary today. I have zero appetite and I just want to go home. The place is starting to depress me - the beeping machines, the hissing of the air con, the once exciting food has become bland, the colourful curtains are boring and I feel so drained. I can barely walk, I go and see the midwife and she promises to send a doctor around but no one turns up. I cry a bit and just to make matters worse, my dear NNU buddy Caz gets the go ahead to go home today. I will be able to move into her big, posh room with a window – at least something. I sit in my chair early afternoon and feed Isla when Rich walks in, what a perfectly timed surprise. He tells me that I look ten years younger now the water retention has passed and it makes me really happy. I still can't believe how much weight I have lost despite my massive intake of chocolate bars and double dinners. He leaves and I take a nap. You really have to take every opportunity to nap, especially when feeling a little low. A nap solves a lot of problems. It's the best medicine ever. Tracey interrupts my nap and tells me that Jess is up and hungry, but it's only been an hour since I last fed her so I talk Tracey into settling her for me which she does. I have dinner and then feed the girls.

I pack all my bags and feel better. Tracey and I make a new plan:

- Jess is ready to go home and can leave tomorrow but we will stay
- if Isla has gained weight by tomorrow we'll reduce top ups
- if Isla gains more weight by Wednesday we'll remove the tube

- exclusively breastfeed both Wednesday and Thursday and have them both in my room

- if Isla has gained weight on Friday we should be able to go home

I am going to stuff my little Isla!

Monday, 26th March

Isla has gained 60 grams. Incredible. The doctor today looks at Isla and decides to drop all top ups. If she gets on well, we'll remove the tube tomorrow. Ellen is in charge today. We give Isla her first bath, totally different to how I expected it to be. We wrap her in a towel and very carefully and briefly wash her head, holding her in a rugby hold, we gently dry her off and then place her on the lower arm, with one hand holding her arm and at the same time supporting her head, hold her above the water, splash her a little and clean the little creases, 60 seconds and that's it. We're done and dry her off and she has a well deserved feed.

I venture out for some food with my boys and realise it's really time to come home; our little outings are becoming more and more difficult. In the evening I decide to take both girls back in my room, what a disaster. They were supposed to be asleep until 11pm but they are both up screaming their heads off and I spend one hour trying to feed them back to sleep on my bed. Isla actually spends from 8pm-11pm at the breast. If they can smell me, they want milk. At 11pm I give up and take them back to the low dependency unit. I sit down to give them a proper feed, one at a time and then pass them to Sarah who settles them within minutes in their cots. This is going to be interesting when we go home as we will definitely be sleeping in the same room for the first six months (as this is recommended in order minimise the risk of cot death). But no time to worry about this now, time is ticking and I need to quickly get some sleep. Feeding and nappy changing now takes around 90 minutes. They feed every three hours, there's actually not much time left to sleep. I need to organise my daytime naps.

Tuesday, 30th March

Jess and Isla are two weeks old today! Jess is discharged today and now also a lodger. Luckily the ward isn't busy and everyone is happy for Jess to stay in a cot next to her sister which is amazing. Isla's tube is removed. Isla passes the car seat test and we hope we can go home tomorrow. I spend most of the day feeding Isla, trying to get as much food as possible into her. The nurse suggests I have them in my room at night as it would make a good impression on the consultant in the morning. I decide to give it another go, by 11:30pm I still haven't slept a minute. Tracey comes to check on me and she takes the girls back to the ward and they settle immediately and we all get two and a half hours sleep. Just before morning Tracey wheels the cots back in my room as if they'd never left. I love her, can I take her home and keep her forever?

Wednesday, 31st March

Isla has lost 14 grams and we are going nowhere. I am so disappointed but at the same time realise that I was expecting too much. The whole day is a bit of a lost day. Jacob and granny come to visit but Jacob is bored of the hospital and they don't stay long. Rich visits in the evening but he is tired. I think we've all had enough of living in two chunks visiting one another. Tonight I am not going to take the girls into my room. My funny dreams return and I wake again without anyone waking me but at least this time at the right time. Tracey is working tonight but is not our nurse, but she keeps coming over to settle Isla for me and I get an okay amount of sleep. Isla restarts the feeding marathon and we decide to try and give her a bottle top up with expressed milk tomorrow night.

Thursday, 1st April

When I get up the world is okay, an hour later I speak to the consultant and everything changes. Yes, it's normal for babies to lose weight when they start breastfeeding, but if you are as little as Isla it really doesn't go down well with consultants. She is talking about replacing the tube unless she gains a substantial amount by tomorrow. Substantial means at least 30 grams. She finishes the conversation with: "I wouldn't pack my bags yet". Thanks for that. She has a point, no, she is right and of course it's all about what's best for Isla but she could have been a little gentler on the sleep deprived emotional wreck that's me.

Jess feeds so well and she is making the funniest faces. Isla is such a determined and steady little muncher. They are both so different and yet so alike. The boys visit briefly. Hopefully this is our last night in here. I pack my bag regardless of any other suggestions.

Friday, 2nd April

We're out of here! Isla has gained enough weight and we can leave. I am so excited! We wrap up the girls, say our "bye byes" and take our little girls out into the real world, to start our real life with two babies and a toddler, without all the wonderful nurses, the milk kitchen and the cooked double dinners. An intense yet very precious time in the neonatal care ward has come to an end and as much as I want to leave, I will miss this place.

A year later

Wow, what a year it's been, I am struggling to believe that my little girls will be one year old tomorrow. We had a lovely day today; Jess and Isla are very happy and healthy. The tiny little baby Isla has grown into a strong and incredibly determined little girl, she doesn't want to miss out on anything. Jess is nearly walking; she is very cheeky and still ever so vocal. I believe their time in my womb has completely shaped their characters, Isla sleeps curled up in a little ball, on her front taking up a tiny amount of space in her big cot. Jess is on her back with arms and legs stretched out far. Isla hoards food in her hands and her cheeks always making sure she gets enough, Jess has one piece at a time and no worries in the world that she might not get enough. I am somewhat sad the first year is already over, it's been the longest, yet shortest year ever and I will miss having two tiny babies but then again I am so excited about the fun times ahead, getting to know my little daughters and move on to teaching them all sorts and to showing my children the world.

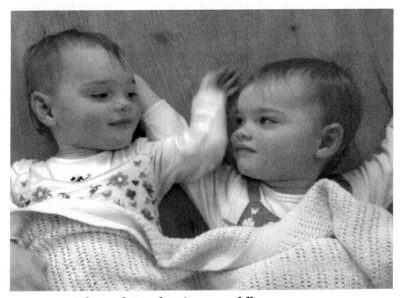

Isla and Jess having a cuddle a year on.

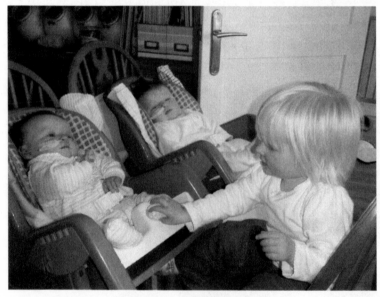

*Big sister Lucy with her
baby twin sisters Sophie and Amy.*

CHAPTER 10

LIFE WITH ADDITIONAL NEEDS

"Family means no one gets left behind or forgotten."
David Ogden Stiers

Sometimes life after birth is different than expected and the challenge of having two babies is combined with the challenges of having additional needs.

Whenever I meet parents of children with additional needs, I notice that what helps them the most appears to be being in touch with other parents in similar situations. It also made me realise that the effects on family life appear to be similar for all of those families, regardless of the particular special need.

I have interviewed two friends of mine, both twin mums, for this chapter and added a few sources of support. I am closing the chapter with a poem written by Emily Perl Kingsley which I find incredibly uplifting.

When you have twins, it quickly becomes apparent if one of them has additional needs, may this be a medical condition, developmental delays, special educational needs or other special needs. When both twins have additional needs the diagnosis can sometimes take longer.

My friend Emma is mum to four year old daughter Lucy and two year old twin girls Amy and Sophie. When I first met Emma at my local multiples club, her twins were newborn babies and my own twins were still tucked up inside my tummy. It was clear that her girls needed extra care as they had problems feeding, but neither Emma nor the health professionals knew what and if there was something unusual with them. It wasn't until Amy and Sophie were over three months old and not smiling that the paediatrician confirmed what Emma had been thinking for a while, that something was indeed unusual.

Emma's husband didn't want to believe it, they'll be just fine. To a certain degree I think he was right because even though they have additional needs they have everything they need, they were born into a loving and caring family, they have one another and their big sister plus a wonderful mother and father. What else do you need as a small child? Emma says that they were incredibly lucky that the girls were eventually diagnosed as there are many special needs children who will never be diagnosed properly. As they are twins she felt they were given more attention which helped, as not only does it help knowing what you are dealing with, it also puts you in the special needs loop and suddenly you're no longer alone. She told me that not knowing what's up with your children makes it incredibly difficult to make plans, especially if you were originally planning to return to work after your maternity leave. You simply need to know where you stand in order to make decisions. Emma's employer was great.

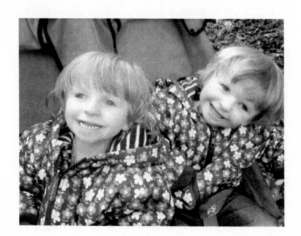

Sophie and Amy having fun on a day out.

When Emma was about to hand in her resignation she suggested for her to take a "career break" and return to work when she was ready.

Emma never told me what her twin girls condition was called, mind you, I didn't ask her either. But once the diagnosis was made, there was a whole new world out there for them.

Emma said: "You just meet some incredible people. You need someone to talk to and you will find that someone. We all seem to have an overwhelming need to talk about our children, we could do a PHD about them, and they are endlessly complex and amazing."

It can be a very emotionally stressful moment when being told, what the diagnosis is and how it will affect family life. The feelings are often described as ranging from disappointment to grief or anger. When I asked Emma how she initially felt about having children with special needs she replied: "I had every possible feeling – some of them very negative. As time went on I became more accepting of the way things were and I fell in love with my girls all over again. Life isn't how we expected it to be and it can be incredibly challenging, however it is also very rewarding and Sophie and Amy light up our lives."

When I asked Emma about the effects on her marriage, she explained that it's hard going through the most difficult thing you've ever been through and at the same time watching someone you dearly love going through it too. "In the early days we tried our best to support one another but sometimes when you feel good about things and positive, your partner might not feel that great and you just don't want to hear about it: I'm alright today, don't bring me down! And this is not being irritable, it's just being pragmatic. But we got used to all this, it's all stages, stages of shock, exhaustion but things became more normal" Emma adds.

Emma's summary of the last two and a half years:

"When they were tiny it was like being sat on a see-saw of feelings going from hugely positive about children and family life to hugely difficult about it all, but with the positive feelings only lasting a few days and the bad ones lasting weeks. By the time the girls were one year I found myself thinking, is this how life is now? At two and a half years life is lovely. They adore each other, they are fun. They are so lucky they have someone just like them. If they weren't twins they might have never met anyone like them. Life is good. The bad times throw you, but they don't last. You've just got to ride with it. When you feel good, enjoy it! There's nothing wrong with enjoying the fact that the baby stage with your children lasts longer, tantrums are delayed, some mums love it that their 15 year olds still snuggle up to them. We got a lot of attention and help and I am enjoying being Sophie and Amy's mum. When times get tough, lower your expectations of yourself, try to get some practical help from family, friends or social services and look after yourself as much as you can while you ride through it. It's about realising that it's all just stages and it won't last forever. Try not to look too far in the future. You don't know what the future holds for any of your children. Try not to concentrate too much on other, older children with the same condition. It will be totally different when your children reach that age as they are your own children and you adore them."

My friend Gemma and her twin daughters Sophie and Heidi plus baby brother Barrett are regulars at my local twins club. I have known the girls since they were first born and gradually the differences in their development became evident. Gemma now shares her story.

SOPHIE'S STORY, written by mum Gemma

My name is Sophie Joy, I am almost three years old and I have Spastic Diplegia Cerebral Palsy (although as we like to say 'I may have Cerebral Palsy, but Cerebral Palsy doesn't have me!') I was born on the 6th of December 2009 with my identical twin sister Heidi. Although I haven't been able to come first with most things due to my disability, I can always say I was the first to enter the world, a whole minute before my sister!! We were born eight weeks early after mummy went into premature labour; we weighed just 4lb 2oz and 4lb 3oz and the first month of our life we spent in the Neonatal Unit at our local hospital, where we also stayed for Christmas! Luckily Father Christmas knew we were there!

The first few months of life at home after NNU were great. We were both doing really well for being born prematurely - feeding well, sleeping well, and crying well! It wasn't until my twin started to do things a lot sooner than me that my family noticed I was a little delayed with my mobility, however this at the time was just put down to developmental delay due to being born prematurely! Ironically for us however, our nana has been a teacher for children with Cerebral Palsy (CP) for years so was able to see the signs of CP in me and my

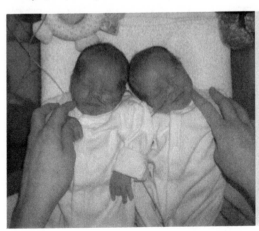

Sophie and Heidi together in Sophie's NNU cot.

mummy and daddy finally pushed for a diagnosis to get me the support I needed! To date, I have had just over a year of physiotherapy to help not only with the tight muscles (spasticity) in my legs, but to install the correct messages to the part of my brain which doesn't work properly, the part that isn't telling my legs to do what they should be doing and climb, walk and run like other children my age do all of the time!

My mummy and daddy have to work hard to keep my physiotherapy up at home and I have had to work tremendously hard just to do simple things such as crawl, kneel up and climb small obstacles. Although I have come on remarkably really, from only being able to commando crawl when I first started physiotherapy at around 1 1/2 years old to now at 2 3/4 years being able to walk using my walker and my family are all extremely proud of the things I have achieved. I still have a long way to go and physiotherapy will be on going for the rest of my life to 'manage' my CP. It will never cure it! Despite this, I am a happy little girl and my family say I always have a smile on my face! I love to play with my friends at nursery, being creative, looking at books, getting messy, being outdoors, everything else any other nearly three year old loves to do! I love the little bit of independence that walking with my frame brings, but the one thing I long to do is to play in the park properly with my twin

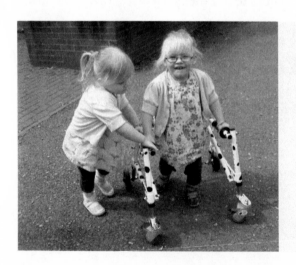

Heidi helping her twin sister Sophie with her walker.

sister Heidi, my big sister Lily and my baby brother Barrett!

Sophie's parents Gemma and Daniel have set up a Just Giving page, please visit their website for more information. www.justgiving.com/stepping-with-sophie

SOURCES OF SUPPORT

In the UK there is Contact a family - www.cafamily.org.uk

This is the UK national charity to support the families of disabled children whatever their condition or disability. "With over 30 years of experience, our vision is that families with disabled children are empowered to live the lives they want and achieve their full potential, for themselves, for the communities they live in, and for society. It's why we offer support, information and advice to over 340,000 families each year and campaign for families to receive a better deal."

This website offers so much. You can enter the diagnosis to find targeted support or get in touch with a family dealing with the same situation or find a local support group.

For other international sources try www.nomotc.org for the US, www.amba.org.au for Australia and www.multiplebirthscanada.org for Canada.

WELCOME TO HOLLAND
BY EMILY PERL KINGSLEY

I am often asked to describe the experience of raising a child
with a disability - to try to help people who have not shared that
unique experience to understand it, to imagine how it would feel.
It's like this......

When you're going to have a baby, it's like planning a fabulous
vacation trip - to Italy. You buy a bunch of guide books and make
your wonderful plans. The Coliseum. The Michelangelo David.
The gondolas in Venice. You may learn some handy phrases in
Italian. It's all very exciting.

After months of eager anticipation, the day finally arrives. You
pack your bags and off you go. Several hours later, the plane
lands. The flight attendant comes in and says,
"Welcome to Holland."
"Holland?!?" you say.
"What do you mean Holland?? I signed up for Italy!
I'm supposed to be in Italy.
All my life I've dreamed of going to Italy."

But there's been a change in the flight plan.
They've landed in Holland and there you must stay.
The important thing is that they haven't taken you to a horrible,
disgusting, filthy place, full of pestilence, famine and disease.
It's just a different place.

So you must go out and buy new guide books. And you must learn a whole new language. And you will meet a whole new group of people you would never have met.

It's just a different place. It's slower-paced than Italy, less flashy than Italy. But after you've been there for a while and you catch your breath, you look around.... and you begin to notice that Holland has windmills....and Holland has tulips. Holland even has Rembrandts.

But everyone you know is busy coming and going from Italy... and they're all bragging about what a wonderful time they had there. And for the rest of your life, you will say "Yes, that's where I was supposed to go. That's what I had planned."

And the pain of that will never, ever, ever, ever go away... because the loss of that dream is a very very significant loss.

But... if you spend your life mourning the fact that you didn't get to Italy, you may never be free to enjoy the very special, the very lovely things ... about Holland.

*   *   *

Emily Perl Kingsley has been a writer for the Sesame Street since 1970. In 1974 her son Jason Kingsley was born with Down Syndrome and inspired her to introduce people with disabilities in the Sesame Street, including an actress who uses a wheelchair and Jason himself. In 1987 she wrote the poem "Welcome to Holland," which has been widely published. Emily Perl Kingsley very kindly granted me permission to include this wonderful poem in my book.

LAST WORDS

Thank you for reading this book. I hope you have enjoyed it and found something for yourself on these pages.

This book was first published as 'Happy Twin Mum' with a different cover and interior design. I initially intended to self publish this book, I formatted the whole book myself, designed the first cover, handed out stacks of proof copies and relied solely on some wonderful, professional people to proof read and give book feedback without charging me.

My children are all still quite young and I have done my best to make this book as helpful as possible. I am sure that one day I will write a revised edition. Therefore any suggestions and feedback, may they be positive or negative, will be greatly received. Please contact me via my website www.lifewithtwins.co.uk.

I wish you and your family
a wonderful, exciting,
happy and healthy life!
Kerri

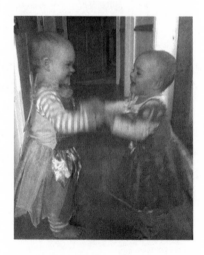

ACKNOWLEDGEMENTS

Thank you to everyone who supported me with this project, especially:

My multiple mum friends around the world for reading the draft and for your photos, stories, feedback and support!

In the UK: Birgitta H., Emma H., Julie W., Maria G., Gemma D., Georgina A., Zoe S., Cassie H., Chloë U., Emma D., Ingrid S., Sarah M., Heidi W., Gill B., Carrie T., Rachael U., Megan H., Tamsin B., Rachael R., Suzie Y., Rachael L., Lindy B., Paula M., Ellen M., Nicky T., Hayley H. Victoria P. and Vicky V.

In Canada: Katy S., Olesea W.

In South Africa: Nicolene M. V., Carmen C.

In the US: Kathryn M. H., Kaycie S. W., Allison B. H.

Theresa B. (Mental Health Nurse) thank you so much for the insights into mental health.

Everyone at Tamba for doing an amazing job and for letting me quote so much Tamba wisdom. www.tamba.org.uk

Cry-Sis for letting me use their checklist. www.cry-sis.org.uk

The Lullaby Trust for letting me include their safer sleep advice and their easy reading cards. www.lullabytrust.org.uk

Bettina Krieger for the beautiful book cover and the illustrations.

Sarah Murray and Laura Burrow for proofing the final copy.

Thank you to my brilliant, honorary readers: Richard B. (Deputy News Editor), Anna T. (Midwife), Carolyn P. (Midwife), Theresa B. (Mental Health Nurse), Helen P.

(General Practitioner), Ann B. (Operational Lead Sure Start Children's Centres), Charlotte L. (Nurse), Sarah N. (Student Nurse), Jennie C. (Teacher), Emma T. (Author), Anita C.S. (Teacher) and Christian C.S. (Journalist).

Kathryn, Emma and Lisa, you are so much more than the world's best babysitters, on many occasions you were my life savers.

My parents-in-law for the invaluable help and the super quick response time during witching-hour dramas.

My parents and my sister for those endless hours of telephone support and all the food and toy deliveries.

And last but not least, a massive thank you to my husband Rich, for enduring four years of book-ramblings. Maybe one day you will actually read this book and find this message. Probably when we're old and wrinkly and digging through some nostalgia. Well, maybe I am being really mean and unfair here, so if you do find this note before the end of 2014 I will wash your van - naked!

ALSO BY KERRI MILLER

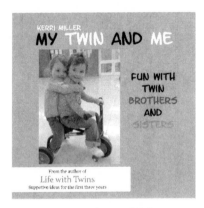

My Twin and Me
by Kerri Miller
ISBN 978-0-9576753-0-8

CPSIA information can be obtained at www.ICGtesting.com
Printed in the USA
BVOW02s1428211215

430732BV00001B/1/P